Blindness and Enlightenment

Blindness and Enlightenment

An Essay

With a new translation of Diderot's *Letter on the Blind* (1749)
and a translation of La Mothe Le Vayer's 'Of a Man-Born-Blind' (1653)

Kate E. Tunstall

continuum

2011

Continuum International Publishing Group
80 Maiden Lane, New York, NY 10038
The Tower Building, 11 York Road, London SE1 7NX

www.continuumbooks.com

Library of Congress Cataloging-in-Publication Data
A catalog record for this book is available from the Library of Congress.

ISBN-13: 978-1-4411-1932-2 (paperback)
ISBN-13: 978-1-4411-5803-1 (hardcover)

Typeset by Pindar NZ, Auckland, New Zealand

Le plus fructueux et naturel exercice de nostre esprit, c'est à mon gré la conference. J'en trouve l'usage plus doux que d'aucune autre action de nostre vie; et c'est la raison pourquoy, si j'estois asture forcé de choisir, je consentirois plustost, ce crois-je, de perdre la veue que l'ouir ou le parler.

[The most fruitful and natural exercise of our mind, in my opinion, is discussion. I find it sweeter than any other action of our life; and that is the reason why, if I were right now forced to choose, I believe I would rather consent to lose my sight than my hearing or speech.]

(Montaigne)

Toute la philosophie n'est fondée que sur deux choses: sur ce qu'on a l'esprit curieux et les yeux mauvais.

[The whole of philosophy is based on two things alone: a curious mind and bad eyesight.]

(Fontenelle)

Tenter de lire [. . .] sans avoir des yeux, c'[est] chercher une épingle avec un gros bâton.

[Trying to read . . . without eyes [is] like looking for a pin with a great big stick.]

(Diderot)

Contents

List of Figures Appearing in the Essay

Acknowledgements

For their conversation, curiosity and insights, I wish to thank Wilda Anderson, Alain Cantillon, Terence Cave, Tim Chesters, Marion Chottin, Andrea Christofidou, Nicholas Cronk, Andrew Curran, Lesel Dawson, Milad Doueihi, Nathalie Ferrand, Finn Fordham, Jim Grant, Marian Hobson, Katherine Ibbett, Anna Kemp, Carl Knappett, Conrad Leyser, Anna Lucas, Patrick Mackie, Thibaut Maus de Rolley, Chris Miller, Ben Morgan, Michael Moriarty, Isabelle Moreau, Jean-Paul Sermain, Joanna Stalnaker, Bernard Sufrin, Alexis Tadié, Rowan Tomlinson, Stephen Williams and Amy Wygant, as well as my family, Pat and Mike Tunstall, Ben Tunstall and Katherine Skellon.

A number of sounding boards gave me very helpful feedback at various stages. I thank, in particular, the Early Modern French Research Seminar (University of Oxford), the Early Modern Seminar (University of London), the research group 'Frontières de la Modernité' (Maison Française d'Oxford), the seminar 'Formes et Idées de la Renaissance aux Lumières' (Paris III-Sorbonne Nouvelle), the Worcester College Women's Research Seminar, and the audience at the session 'In and Around the *Encyclopédie*' (French Studies, Oxford).

The University of Oxford provides an ideal environment in which to think, talk and write, and Worcester College has sustained me in these and other no less essential ways: I am particularly grateful to the Senior Common Room staff, Neil Turner, Asia Twardowska and Paula Wallbridge, for allowing me last-minute lunches, and to the Head Gardener, Simon Bagnall, and his team for creating an amazing 'spectacle of nature' in the College gardens. Other support, moral as well as technical and administrative, was provided by Cath Fraser, Jane Gover, Karen James, Marilyn Peddie, Elizabeth Smith and Emma Standhaft.

It was my extraordinary good fortune to have a team of readers to guide me through what I had written when I could no longer see it clearly and to suggest signposts, alternative routes and short cuts. I wish to thank Emma Herdman for her remarkable tact and eagle eyes, Richard Scholar for his terrifically helpful 'pesky squiggles' and his willingness to debate them at short notice, Caroline Warman for her exceptional generosity of ideas and for knowing when things are funny (and when they're not), and

Wes Williams for his fine-tuned ear for echoes and rhythms, or perhaps that should be rhythms and echoes. My greatest debts are to Alain, his one-eyed horse and *le virage Viala*.

Oxford and Saint Affrique (Aveyron), 2010

Some of the material appearing in Chapters 1, 2 and 6 has appeared elsewhere as "'Des circonstances assez peu philosophiques': Diderot's 'aveugle-né du Puiseaux'" in *French Studies Bulletin*, 99 (2006), 33–6; 'The Judgement of Experience: Reading and Seeing in Diderot's *Lettre sur les aveugles*' in *French Studies*, 62.4 (2008), 404–16; 'Pré-histoire d'un emblème des Lumières: l'aveugle-né de Montaigne à Diderot', in Isabelle Moreau (ed.), *Les Lumières en mouvement: la circulation des idées au XVIIIe siècle* (Lyon: ENS, 2009), pp. 173–97; 'L'Aveugle qui suit l'aveugle qui suit l'aveugle: la philosophie intertextuelle de la *Lettre sur les aveugles*' in Marion Chottin (ed.), *L'Aveugle et le philosophe* (Paris: Presses Universitaires de Paris-Sorbonne, 2009), pp. 63–81; and 'Philosophy, Ethics and the Work of Fiction', Alexis Tadié and Richard Scholar (eds), *Fiction and the Frontiers of Knowledge in Europe, 1500–1800* (Aldershot: Ashgate, 2011), pp. 107–21.

Note on the References

References are made to two French editions of the *Lettre sur les aveugles.* The first reference is to the standard scholarly edition in volume 4 of Denis Diderot, *Œuvres complètes,* Herbert Dieckmann, Jacques Proust and Jean Varloot (eds), 30+ volumes (Paris: Hermann, 1975–). The second is to the paperback edition in Denis Diderot, *Lettre sur les aveugles. Lettre sur les sourds et muets,* Marian Hobson and Simon Harvey (eds), (Paris: Garnier-Flammarion, 2000), pp. 28–86. The first is referred to as 'DPV, 4', the second as 'Hobson and Harvey'. All references to the *Letter on the Blind* (referred to as 'the *Letter*') are to my English translation, found here in the Appendix, pp. 167–227.

For other non-English language texts, the first reference gives the original title, followed by the English title or translation in square brackets; subsequent references give only the original title. All translations, unless otherwise stated, are mine.

Prologue, or Operation Enlightenment

One Saturday, I open the newspaper to find inside a leaflet from a charitable organisation requesting a donation. On the cover, it shows a picture of a child with cloudy eyes: he is suffering from cataracts. I open the leaflet and my eyes are drawn to the following testimony:

> I took the bandage off his eyes. The young boy looked around and then looked at his mother. There was silence for a moment, then he said something to her. She burst into tears, and so did the boy. I ran to get a translator as worried thoughts flashed through my mind . . .
>
> The translator slowly turned to me and said, 'Don't worry.' The child had told his mother that this was the first time he could see her. He said she was beautiful.[1]

Beneath it, we see the boy, now smiling, his eyes bright, and a direct debit form.

The story of the first moments of sight that culminates in a moving recognition scene may of course be authentic, but it also belongs to a genre with a long history. This sentimental narrative involving a travelling cataract surgeon, a post-operative cataract patient and his mother, is likely to strike any reader familiar with Enlightenment and eighteenth-century writing as remarkably similar to the accounts of cataract operations that were published in the press three hundred years ago.

In 1709, for example, the London magazine *Tatler* published an account of a cataract operation performed by the itinerant oculist, Roger Grant, on a young man by the name of William Jones from Newington Butts in Surrey. It related the following:

> When the Patient first receiv'd the Dawn of Light, there appear'd such an Ecstasy in his Action that he seemed ready to swoon away in the Surprise of Joy and Wonder . . . When he had continued in this Amazement some Time, his Mother could no longer bear the

1 ORBIS Saving Sight Worldwide.

> Agitations of so many Passions as throng'd upon her; but fell upon his Neck, crying out, 'My Son! My Son!' The Youth knew her Voice, and could speak no more than, 'Oh me! Are You my Mother?' and fainted.[2]

The story is, we are told, 'proper at once to exercise our Humanity, please our Imaginations, and improve our Judgements'.[3] More than seventy years later, in 1782, a similar story would be told about the French oculist, Jacques Daviel:

> La bienfaisance de Daviel conduisait, de toutes les provinces du royaume dans son laboratoire, des malades indigents qui venaient implorer son secours, et sa réputation y appelait une assemblée curieuse, instruite et nombreuse. Je crois que nous en faisions partie le même jour, M. Marmontel et moi. Le malade était assis; voilà sa cataracte enlevée; Daviel pose sa main sur des yeux qui venaient de rouvrir à la lumière. Une femme âgée, debout à côté de lui, montrait le plus vif intérêt au succès de l'opération; elle tremblait de tous ses membres à chaque mouvement de l'opérateur. Celui-ci lui fait signe d'approcher, et la place à genoux en face de l'opéré; il éloigne ses mains, le malade ouvre les yeux, il voit, il s'écrie: Ah! c'est ma mère! . . . Je n'ai jamais entendu un cri plus pathétique; il me semble que je l'entends encore. La vieille femme s'évanouit, les larmes coulent des yeux des assistants, et les aumônes tombent de leurs bourses.[4]
>
> Daviel's good works led the indigent sick to come from every province of the kingdom to his operating room to beg for his help, and his reputation brought in a wide, learned and curious public. I think Marmontel and I were there on the same day. The patient was seated; now the cataract is removed, and Daviel places his hands over the eyes that were just re-opened to the light. An elderly woman standing next to him was showing the liveliest of interests in the success of operation; she was shaking all over at the surgeon's every move. He gestures to her to come close and makes her kneel in front of the patient; he removes his hands and the patient opens his eyes; he can see and cries out: Ah! You're my mother! . . . I have never heard such a pathetic cry; it's as though I can still hear it. The

---

2 *Tatler*, 55 (Tuesday, August 16, 1709), in *The Tatler*, Donald F. Bond (ed.), 3 volumes (Oxford: Clarendon Press, 1987), vol. 1, pp. 384–5.

3 *Tatler*, 55, p. 384.

4 *Additions à la Lettre sur les aveugles* [Additions to the Letter on the Blind], in Hobson and Harvey, pp. 247–8.

old lady passes out, tears flow from the eyes of all those present, and alms from their purses.

There are, of course, differences between these narratives and that found in the twenty-first-century charity leaflet. Whereas in the modern narrative the surgeon misreads the tears of the African boy and his mother, here there is no room for misunderstanding and no need for translators as the emotional response of the spectators is as legible as the vocabulary is melodramatic: the *Tatler* journalist refers to the 'dawn of sight' and says William Jones' mood is of 'ecstasy', and Marmontel's companion's ears are still ringing with the cry.

Indeed, emotions run so high in the eighteenth century that someone almost always passes out, which may lead us to suspect the stories of parody. Certainly, the one in *Tatler* was itself the object of parody – the *Female Tatler* quipped 'Happy are they that can see to read it!';[5] and the reference to Marmontel, a writer well known for moral tales, hints that the story might be, if not quite parody, then certainly pastiche. Of course, the ingenuous little tale in the modern charity leaflet might also be pastiched and parodied, though I suspect that a reader unfamiliar with its eighteenth-century antecedents is likely to censor any such thought owing to the organisation's charitable motives.

The relationship between the narratives and the request for money is also handled rather differently. While *The Spectator* later assures its readers that 'many who could not purchase [Grant's] Assistance with Money, have enjoy'd it from his Charity',[6] the economic motives underlying Daviel's performing his operation in public are brought out in the comparison between tears and alms (and we should note his use of the term 'interests' with its emotional and economic connotations).[7] As for the modern leaflet, its detachable direct debit form makes its aims perfectly clear.

Such differences aside, however, all three cataract narratives present the recovery of sight as a coming back to life. They occlude any possibility that the patient might feel any pain – less a possibility than a certainty in the eighteenth century; and they describe a joyful experience of rebirth in which, this time round, sons recognize their mothers. To see is, these stories suggest, not only to be alive, but also to know oneself to be so.

5 *Female Tatler* (15 November 1709) in Bernard Mandeville, *By a Society of Ladies: Essays in The Female Tatler*, M. M. Goldsmith (ed.) (Bristol: Thoemmes, 1999), p. 88.

6 *The Spectator*, 472 (Monday, 1 September 1712), in *The Spectator*, Donald F. Bond (ed.), 5 volumes (Oxford: Clarendon Press, 1965), vol. 4, p. 173.

7 See Alain Viala, *Lettre à Rousseau sur l'intérêt littéraire* (Paris: Presses Universitaires de France, 2005), pp. 108–26.

Misrecognition Scenes

Not all accounts of the first moments of sight involve an emotional spectacle of recognition, however. Some stage scenes of misrecognition that have philosophical and scientific implications. In 1688, in a trailer for his *Essay Concerning Human Understanding*, which would be published in 1690, Locke observed that a man who had been blind since birth could have no idea of colour; but could he have an idea of shape and, if so, would it be the same idea as the one a sighted person has? This was the question put to Locke by the Irish philosopher, William Molyneux, in the form of the following thought-experiment:

> Suppose a Man born blind, and now adult, and taught by his touch to distinguish between a Cube and a Sphere of the same metal, and nighly of the same bigness, so as to tell, when he felt one and t'other, which is the Cube, which is the Sphere. Suppose then the Cube and Sphere placed on a Table, and the Blind Man made to see. *Quaere*, Whether by his sight, before he touch'd them, he could now distinguish, and tell, which is the Globe, which the Cube.[8]

Molyneux's Problem, as it came to be known, involving a man who had been born blind suddenly being able to see – a purely hypothetical scenario as the repeated imperative 'suppose' and the man's rather sudden acquisition of sight suggest – was designed to investigate whether the idea of shape gained through the sense of touch is the same as the idea of shape gained through sight. Locke took up the problem in the second edition of his *Essay* (1694) and, for reasons that we shall examine later but which are related to his refutation of Cartesian science, he said that, 'the Blind Man, at first sight, would not be able with certainty to say which was the Globe, which the Cube, whilst he only saw them; though he could unerringly name them by his touch, and certainly distinguish them by the difference of their Figures felt'.[9] The success of Locke's *Essay*, combined no doubt with the puzzling appeal of the thought-experiment, meant that Molyneux's Problem would hold the attention of several generations of philosophers across Europe – Leibniz, Berkeley, Voltaire, La Mettrie, Maupertuis, Condillac, Turgot, Diderot,

8 *The Correspondence of John Locke*, E.S. de Beer (ed.), 9 volumes (Oxford: Clarendon Press, 1976–89), vol. 3, no. 1064, pp. 482–3. Locke did not reply. Molyneux's second letter, which again posed the question, is dated 2 March 1693, *The Correspondence of John Locke*, vol. 4, no. 1609, pp. 647–52. See also John Locke, *An Essay Concerning Human Understanding*, Peter H. Nidditch (ed. and foreword) (Oxford: Oxford University Press, 1979), p. 146.

9 Locke, *Essay*, p. 146.

Mérian, Reid, to name but the most famous.[10]

It did not, however, remain a thought-experiment for long. If, in 1709, Berkeley merely speculated as to whether Grant and his patients could provide some data that would solve the problem empirically,[11] in 1727, an apparently reliable source was found: a boy who had been born blind but whose cataracts had been successfully removed by the surgeon and Fellow of the Royal Society, William Cheselden. Cheselden reported in the *Philosophical Transactions of the Royal Society* that the boy, at first sight and indeed for some time following his operation, could not recognize shapes. Cheselden narrates a misrecognition scene in which the boy fails to recognize, not his mother, but his household pets:

> When he first saw . . . he knew not the Shape of any Thing, nor any one Thing from another, however different in Shape, or Magnitude; but upon being told what Things were, whose Form he before knew from feeling, he would carefully observe, that he might know them again; but having too many Objects to learn at once, he forgot many of them; and (as he said) at first he learn'd to know, and again forgot a thousand Things in a Day. One Particular only (though it may appear trifling) I will relate; Having often forgot which was the Cat and which the Dog, he was asham'd to ask; but catching the Cat (which he knew by feeling) he was observ'd to look at her stedfastly, and then setting her down, said, So Puss! I shall know you another Time.[12]

The detail of the cat and the dog may appear 'trifling', but in fact, as Cheselden well knew – and indeed as his calling attention to its apparent triflingness and the rhythm of his sentence both suggest – the boy's failure to recognize 'which was the Cat and which the Dog' answered the question of 'which is the Globe, which the Cube'. And so it seemed that knowledge about the workings of the human mind could be gained by observing an ex-blind man nonetheless failing to see; indeed it became, as Foucault has influentially described it, one of the Enlightenment's foundational myths. He says of the period:

---

10 Kant's absence from this list has been explored by Brigitte Sassen in 'Kant on Molyneux's Problem'. *British Journal for the History of Philosophy* 12.3 (2004), 471–85.

11 George Berkeley, *New Theory of Vision*, second edition (Dublin: Printed by Aaron Rhames for Jeremy Pepyat, 1709), pp. 197–98.

12 'An Account of some Observations Made by a Young Gentleman, Who Was Born Blind, or Lost His Sight so Early, That He Had no Remembrance of Ever Having Seen, and Was Couch'd Between 13 and 14 Years of Age'. *Philosophical Transactions of the Royal Society*, vol. 35 (1727–1728) (London: W. Innys, 1665–1886), pp. 447–50.

> L'enfance, la jeunesse des choses et des hommes étaient chargées d'un pouvoir ambigu: dire la naissance de la vérité; mais aussi mettre à l'épreuve la vérité tardive des hommes, la rectifier, la rapprocher de sa nudité . . . Inlassablement, en chaque enfant, les choses répètent leur jeunesse, le monde reprend contact avec sa forme natale: il n'est jamais adulte pour qui le regarde pour la première fois. Quand il a dénoué ses parentés vieillies, l'œil peut s'ouvrir au ras des choses et des âges; et de tous les sens et de tous les savoirs, il a l'habileté de pouvoir être le plus malhabile en répétant agilement sa lointaine ignorance . . . L'oreille a ses préférences, la main ses traces et ses plis; l'œil, qui a parenté avec la lumière, ne supporte que son présent. Ce qui permet à l'homme de renouer avec l'enfance et de rejoindre la permanente naissance de la vérité, c'est cette naïveté claire, distante, ouverte du regard. D'où les deux grandes expériences mythiques où la philosophie du XVIIIe siècle a voulu fonder son commencement: le spectateur étranger dans un pays inconnu et l'aveugle de naissance rendu à la lumière.[13]

> Childhood, the youth of things and of men were endowed with an ambiguous power: to tell of the birth of truth, but also to put to the test older men's truth, to rectify it, bring it closer to its nakedness . . . In every child, things tirelessly speak their youth, the world resumes contact with its native form; it is never adult to someone who sees it for the first time. When it has untied its old bonds of kinship, the eye can peel away layers and generations; and of all the senses and all the sources of knowledge, it is has the skill of seeming unskilled as it nimbly renews its distant ignorance . . . The ear has its preferences, the hand its lines and folds; the eye, in kinship with light, bears only its present. What allows man to resume contact with childhood and rediscover the permanent birth of truth is this bright, distant, open naïvety of the gaze. Hence the two great mythical experiences on which the philosophy of the eighteenth century wished to found its beginning: the foreign spectator in an unknown country and the man-born-blind restored to the light.[14]

---

13 Michel Foucault, *Naissance de la clinique* (Paris: Presses Universitaires de France, 1963), pp. 63–4.

14 Michael Foucault, *The Birth of the Clinic*, A. M. Sheridan (trans.) (London: Tavistock, 1973), pp. 64–65 (translation significantly modified).

Molyneux's Problem has not gone away; it continues to be debated.[15] And Cheselden's report inaugurated a tradition of failed recognition narratives that continues to this day, though the discipline concerned now tends to be popular neuroscience rather than empiricist epistemology. In 'To See and not See' (1991), Oliver Sacks, the neuroscientist probably most famous for his collection of essays, *The Man who Mistook his Wife for a Hat* (1985), tells the following story:

> Amy and Virgil would be getting married soon – wouldn't it be fantastic if he could see? If, after a near-lifetime of blindness, his first vision could be his bride, the wedding, the minister, the church! Dr. Hamlin had agreed to operate, and the cataract on Virgil's right eye had been removed a fortnight earlier, Amy's father informed me. And, miraculously, the operation had worked. Amy, who began keeping a journal the day after the operation – the day the bandages were removed – wrote in her initial entry: 'Virgil can SEE! . . . Entire office in tears, first time Virgil has sight for forty years . . . Virgil's family so excited, crying, can't believe it! . . . Miracle of sight restored incredible!' . . . Virgil told me later that in this first moment he had no idea what he was seeing. There was light, there was movement, there was color, all mixed up, all meaningless, a blur. Then out of the blur came a voice that said, 'Well?' Then, and only then, he said, did he finally realize that this chaos of light and shadow was a face – and, indeed, the face of his surgeon.[16]

While Amy's testimony belongs to the sentimental genre of the *Tatler*, Sacks' framing narrative and its counter-testimony of Virgil's failed recognition recall Cheselden's report of nearly three hundred years earlier.

The story of the first moments of sight, whether recounted for charitable, moral, comic, philosophical or neurological purposes, is a privileged narrative topos because it is overloaded with symbolic significance. As numerous studies have shown,[17] visual metaphors are massively present in Western culture from the Greeks to the Enlightenment and beyond, and notably in Christianity. Knowledge, truth and faith are commonly presented in terms of sight and light. Martin Jay has demonstrated as

---

15 For recent discussions, see, for example, Laura Berchielli, 'Colour, Space and Figure in Locke: An Interpretation of the Molyneux Problem'. *Journal of the History of Philosophy*, 40.1 (2002), pp. 47–65; Janet Levin, 'Molyneux's Question and the Individuation of Perceptual Concepts'. *Philosophical Studies*, 139 (2008), pp. 1–28.

16 Oliver Sacks, *An Anthropologist on Mars* (New York: Vintage, 1995), pp. 108–9.

17 See, for example, Teresa Brennan and Martin Jay, *Vision in Context: Historical and Contemporary Perspectives on Sight* (London: Routledge, 1996).

much in the opening paragraph to his history of vision, *Downcast Eyes* (1994), which contains twenty-one visual metaphors:

> Even a rapid glance at the language we commonly use will demonstrate the ubiquity of visual metaphors. If we actively focus our attention on them vigilantly keeping an eye out for those deeply embedded as well as those on the surface, we can gain an illuminating insight into the complex mirroring of perception and language. Depending, of course, on one's point of view or outlook, the prevalence of such metaphors will be counted an obstacle or an aid to our knowledge of reality. It is, however, no idle speculation or figment of the imagination to claim that if blinded to their importance, we will damage our ability to inspect the world outside and introspect the world within. And our prospects for escaping their thrall, if indeed that is a foreseeable goal, will be greatly dimmed. In lieu of an exhaustive survey of such metaphors, whose scope is far too broad to allow an easy synopsis, this opening paragraph should suggest how ineluctable the modality of the visual actually is, at least in our linguistic practice. I hope by now that you, *optique lecteur*, can see what I mean.[18]

In the cataract narratives, sight may be literal, but its metaphorical counterparts of truth, reason, knowledge and faith are never far away. Close to hand too are the various stories of Christ healing the blind man – the most famous of the miracles recounted in the New Testament. The Gospel of St Mark, for example, relates:

> And he cometh to Bethsaida; and they bring a blind man unto him, and besought him to touch him. And he took the blind man by the hand, and led him out of the town; and when he had spit on his eyes, and put his hands upon him, he asked him if he saw ought. And he looked up, and said, I see men as trees, walking. After that he put *his* hands again upon his eyes, and made him look up: and he was restored, and saw every man clearly.[19]

---

18 Martin Jay, *Downcast Eyes: The Denigration of Vision in Twentieth-Century French Thought* (Berkeley: University of California Press, 1994), p. 1. He explains in a footnote: '*vigilant* is derived from the Latin *vigilare*, to watch, which in its French form *veiller* is the root of *surveillance*. *Demonstrate* comes from the Latin *monstrare*, to show. *Inspect, prospect, introspect* (and other words like *aspect* and *circumspect*) all derive from the Latin *specere*, to look at or observe. *Speculate* has the same root. *Scope* comes from the Latin *scopium*, a translation of a Greek word for to look at or examine. *Synopsis* is from the Greek word for general view' (p. 1, note 1).

19 Mark 8.22-25. All references are to the King James Bible.

This story and others like it from the Christian tradition resonate in the cataract narratives, creating a sense that the surgeon has performed something akin to a miracle, conferred more than just the physical sense of sight on the patient who has come not only to see but also to see 'the light'.

Scene Unseen

The 1782 pastiche of the morally uplifting and financially rewarding recognition scene, quoted earlier, forms one of the 'Additions' to a work published anonymously over thirty years previously, entitled *Lettre sur les aveugles à l'usage de ceux qui voient* [Letter on the Blind for the Use of Those Who Can See] (1749).[20] The author was Diderot.

Denis Diderot (1713–1784) would later be known primarily for his role as co-editor of the *Encyclopédie* [Encyclopædia] (1751–1772), the major publishing event of the Enlightenment, which defined – both in its pages and as a result of the controversies and quarrels surrounding it – the eighteenth-century *philosophe* as a writer committed to disseminating knowledge, conceived of in rational, scientific and secular terms. As a *philosophe*, Diderot would write for the theatre, both plays and dramatic theory, and he would write, but not publish, works of art criticism, comic novels and dialogues, and observations on, supplements to and refutations of numerous works by his contemporaries, exploring a wide range of philosophical, æsthetic, moral and ethical questions. But in late May or early June 1749 when the *Letter on the Blind* first appeared,[21] Diderot's reputation as a *philosophe* had not yet been made; the *Letter* would play a significant role in its making.

The *Letter* is an important intervention in the debates that Molyneux's Problem was continuing to provoke in France in the 1740s, and the intervention it makes is also highly unusual: rather than taking the form of a discussion in a philosophical essay, as it does in Locke or

---

20 In addition to withholding the name of the author, the title page also withholds that of the publisher, though it gives a place of publication, namely, London. In fact, the *Letter* was published in Paris, printed by Pierre-Guillaume Simon, and distributed by Laurent Durand, one of the most important booksellers and publishers in eighteenth-century Paris; and he did so illegally – the *Letter* has no 'privilège', which is to say that Durand had not been granted permission to make it available to the public. For more information, see Frank A. Kafker and Jeff Loveland, 'The Elusive Laurent Durand, a Leading Publisher of the French Enlightenment'. *SVEC*, 12 (2005), 223–58, and 'Diderot et Laurent Durand, son éditeur principal'. *Recherches sur Diderot et l'Encyclopédie*, 39 (2005), 29–40. For a history of 'privilèges' and permissions, see Roger Chartier, *The Cultural Origins of the French Revolution*, Lydia G. Cochrane (trans.) (Durham, NC: Duke University Press, 1991), especially the chapter, 'The Way of Print', pp. 38–67.

21 See Anne-Marie Chouillet, 'Trois lettres inédites de Diderot'. *Recherches sur Diderot et l'Encyclopédie*, 11 (1991), 10–17, p. 10.

Condillac, it takes that of a fictitious piece of correspondence, written by an unnamed man to a woman he calls simply 'Madame'. In it he postpones for as long as possible any scene of post-operative philosophical misrecognition and denies her any scene of joyful recognition, even as he acknowledges that such scenes were what she had been hoping for. Instead the *Letter* presents its reader with two men, both born blind and neither with any prospect of seeing. Their inoperable state presents little cause for despair, however, as one of the men-born-blind has no desire to see and the other, the Chair in Mathematics at the University of Cambridge, has no need to. Together, they suggest that sight may not be all it is cracked up to be and that blindness is not necessarily the inferior and pitiful state of deprivation the sighted tend to think it is and therefore wish to cure. Most provocatively, their testimony calls into question the interest and value of any spectacle of revelation – literal or metaphorical. It is this complex and contrarian work that is the object of this book.

For those readers who are unfamiliar with the *Letter*, a brief summary of it will be helpful here. It has a loose conversational structure, common in the epistolary form, but in which we can identify five sections,[22] each one generically different.

A short prologue is followed by a narrative that recounts a visit to the home of 'l'aveugle-né du Puiseaux' [the man-born-blind of Puiseaux] and tells of his blind way of life and, amongst other things, what he thinks about sight and the sighted. This leads into a third section, the central concern of which is the sense of touch: it begins with a speculative exploration of the differences between how the sighted and the blind think, and ends with a highly pedagogical explanation, accompanied by a series of visual plates, of the way in which the blind Cambridge mathematician, Nicholas Saunderson, did complex calculations by palpable means.

The most well-known part of the *Letter* follows this: it is a conversation between Saunderson, who is approaching death, and his sighted vicar, Gervaise Holmes, in which the blind man contests Holmes's belief in God on the grounds that it relies on the wondrous spectacle of nature, which he cannot see. In Saunderson's view, there is no such thing as intelligent design and nature operates instead in an entirely random way; it is, in short, blind. This is not only the best-known part of the *Letter*, but the views that Saunderson expresses in it are also generally taken to be the main point of the whole text.

In the final part, the *Letter* enters a philosophical discussion of Molyneux's Problem and of its various existing solutions, proposes

22 Hobson and Harvey identify only three sections; see Hobson and Harvey, p. 11.

another, and ends on a series of questions regarding the limited state and, perhaps, limited nature of human knowledge. The *Letter* also has a number of paratextual features, an epigraph, two footnotes and an index, which are every bit as important as the rest of the text.

Introduction

Optics and Tactics

In the twentieth century, many French writers and philosophers – Bergson, Bataille, Merleau-Ponty, Foucault and Derrida – took a critical interest in the predominance of visual metaphors in Western thought and sought both to expose the assumptions such metaphors foster and to counter them by focusing instead on visual dysfunction, including blindness, and on the other senses, notably touch.[1] In light of their work, Diderot's *Letter on the Blind* has come to appear visionary.

A number of recent histories of vision and visuality, of blindness and touch, position the *Letter* as a point of origin for this critical re-evaluation of blindness and the blind, and for the hostility to vision that they take to be a hallmark of much modern and post-modern thought. The most influential argument of this kind has been made by Martin Jay, whose *Downcast Eyes* (1994) was quoted earlier. For Jay, Diderot's *Letter* anticipates the twentieth-century critique of what he calls the 'ancien scopic régime.'[2] Its interest in blindness is read as a challenge to Cartesian perspectivalism and its investigation of touch as proto-phenomenological.[3] For the literary critic, William Paulson, in *Enlightenment, Romanticism and the Blind in France* (1987), the *Letter* looks forward to the Romantic reinvestment with insight and beyond that, to Foucault's analyses of the social and historical construction of illness.[4] From the perspective of a social historian also, that of Zina Weygand in *The Blind in French Society from the Middle Ages to the Century of Louis Braille* (2009), the *Letter* represents a definitive turn away from a medieval and early modern view of the blind as social outcasts and a key move in the modern treatment of the

1 For an overview, see Jay, *Downcast Eyes*, pp. 149–435.

2 Jay, *Downcast Eyes*, pp. 149–210.

3 Jay, *Downcast Eyes*, p. 103. See also Mark Paterson, *The Senses of Touch: Haptics, Affects and Technologies* (Oxford: Berg, 2007), p. 47.

4 William R. Paulson, *Enlightenment, Romanticism and the Blind in France* (Princeton: Princeton University Press, 1987). See also Edward Larrissy, *The Blind and Blindness in Literature of the Romantic Period* (Edinburgh: Edinburgh University Press, 2007), and Simon Hayhoe, *God, Money, and Politics: English Attitudes to Blindness and Touch, from the Enlightenment to Integration* (Charlotte: Information Age Publishing, 2008).

blind as equal members of society, possessing dignity and rights.[5]

This essay tells a different kind of story about the *Letter* and its relationship to the history of vision and blindness. Instead of reading the *Letter* as a point of origin for a modern or post-modern critique of a pre-modern ocularcentric vision of blindness, I argue for a greater sense of continuity with earlier texts. I show the ways in which the *Letter* mobilizes the comic figure of the blind man, found in much early modern culture, and, more importantly, the extent to which it exploits the figure of the man who has been blind since birth, and who is to be found in early modern scepticism. This is a philosophical and literary tradition that has been almost entirely overlooked in histories of vision. As Stuart Clark has observed in *Vanities of the Eye* (2007), which challenges Jay's account of the hegemony of vision in early modern France, scepticism with its doubting attitude to knowledge gained on the basis of the evidence of the senses meant that writers and thinkers in the early modern period 'lost their optical nerve.'[6] This essay argues that such a loss of nerve brings the blind into view and shows that blind men or, more accurately, men-born-blind make regular and significant appearances in sceptical texts. They can be found in the work of numerous early modern French philosophers and writers, such as Montaigne, Charron, Gassendi, La Mothe Le Vayer and Cyrano de Bergerac. Each takes their cue, albeit in different ways, from Sextus Empiricus, whose *Outlines of Scepticism* was the major stimulus for sceptical thought in the early modern period.[7] The relationships between these men-born-blind and those of the *Letter* have not been accorded any sustained attention by critics.[8] I trace them here, showing them to be at

5 Zina Weygand, *The Blind in French Society from the Middle Ages to the Century of Louis Braille* (Stanford: Stanford University Press, 2009), p. 7. Such rights would be formalized in the creation of the Institute for Blind Youth in 1785, which was nationalized by the Constituent Assembly in 1791.

6 Stuart Clark, *Vanities of the Eye: Vision in Early Modern European Culture* (Oxford: Oxford University Press, 2007), p. 2.

7 See Luciano Floridi, *Sextus Empiricus: The Transmission and Recovery of Pyrrhonism* (Oxford: Oxford University Press, 2002); Richard H. Popkin, *The History of Scepticism: From Savonarola to Bayle*, revised and expanded edition (Oxford: Oxford University Press, 2003); José R. Maia Neto and Richard H. Popkin (eds), *Skepticism in Renaissance and Post-Renaissance Thought: New Interpretations* (New York: Humanity Books, 2004).

8 Jerome Schwartz and Francine Markovits are notable exceptions. See Jerome Schwartz, *Diderot and Montaigne. The Essais and the Shaping of Diderot's Humanism* (Geneva: Droz, 1966); Francine Markovits, 'L'aveugle, une figure de la philosophie sceptique'. *VOIR*, 19 (1999), 34–51. By contrast, Jean-Claude Bourdin has asserted that 'on chercherait en vain dans son œuvre l'exploitation des "lieux communs" sceptiques' [Diderot was doubtless never a sceptic and we would search his work in vain for the use of sceptical 'commonplaces'] ('Matérialisme et scepticisme chez Diderot'. *Recherches sur Diderot et l'Encyclopédie*, 26 (1999), 85–97, p. 85).

once philosophical and literary, and arguing that the *Letter* as a whole produces many of its meanings in relation to these intertexts.

The *Letter* is usually said to have an obvious atheist and materialist meaning, and to belong to what is increasingly being called the 'radical Enlightenment'.[9] The most widely available edition of Diderot's complete works, that edited by Laurent Versini, presents the *Letter* as 'le premier manifeste éclatant de sa philosophie originale, c'est-à-dire de son athéisme et de son matérialisme biologique'. [the first explosive manifesto of his original philosophy, that is, of his atheism and his biological materialism].[10] For my purposes here, what is important about this claim is not Versini's use of the adjective 'biological' to describe materialism, which has been disputed by a number of critics who have offered a wide range of alternatives;[11] rather it is his concern to establish the *Letter* as a work manifestly written by an atheist and a materialist, and as a turning point within Diderot's intellectual development which prepared the ground for his later unpublished works on the body, notably *Le Rêve de d'Alembert* [D'Alembert's Dream] (1769) and the *Eléments de physiologie* [Elements of Physiology] (1773–4). Similar claims about the philosophical message of the *Letter* that also situate it in the wider context of the French Enlightenment can be found in intellectual history. Jonathan Israel's *Radical Enlightenment* (2001), for instance, accords the *Letter*, along with La Mettrie's *L'Homme Machine* [Machine Man] (1748), a pre-eminent place in mid eighteenth-century atheist, materialist thought.[12] It cites, as almost all critics and editors do, the fact that Diderot was arrested shortly after its publication as evidence of its particularly subversive content.[13]

All four aspects of these claims – that the *Letter* presents a clear break from Diderot's earlier work, that it has a manifestly atheist and materialist message, that such atheism and materialism can be taken to be Diderot's, and that his arrest confirms any of the previous claims – need examination.

---

9 See Margaret Jacob, *Radical Enlightenment: Pantheists, Freemasons and Republicans* (London and Boston: George Allen and Unwin, 1981); Jonathan Israel, *Radical Enlightenment: Philosophy and the Making of Modernity, 1650–1750* (Oxford: Oxford University Press, 2001).

10 Denis Diderot, *Œuvres*, Laurent Versini (ed.), 5 volumes (Paris: Laffont, 1994–7), vol. 1, p. 135.

11 See Jean-Claude Bourdin, *Diderot. Le matérialisme* (Paris: Presses Universitaires de France, 1998), p. 13.

12 Israel, *Radical Enlightenment*, p. 710.

13 Israel, *Radical Enlightenment*, p. 710. See also Hobson and Harvey, p. 7.

*****, or the letter-writer formerly known as 'Diderot'**

While critics have given some attention to the possible identity of the *Letter*'s addressee, referred to in the text simply as 'Madame', no serious consideration has been given to the man who addresses her. It has been observed that 'Madame' might be a real person – perhaps Diderot's mistress, Madame de Puisieux, whom he had met in 1745,[14] or perhaps the mathematician, Madame de Prémontval, to whom Diderot may have addressed his *Mémoires sur différents sujets de mathématiques* [Memoirs on different subjects in mathematics] (1748).[15] She might, instead, be a wholly fictitious persona, akin, though socially inferior, to the Marquise in Fontenelle's *Entretiens sur la pluralité des mondes* [Conversations on the Plurality of Worlds] (1686).[16]

The first-person pronoun, 'je' [I], which addresses Madame, has posed readers no such difficulties, however; 'I' has simply been assumed to be Diderot, the writer of the *Letter*. Such an assumption has, perhaps somewhat paradoxically, been aided rather than obstructed by the fact that the original publication was anonymous. The *Letter* is signed 'Votre très humble et très obéissant serviteur, ***' [Your most humble and most obedient servant, ***].[17] Clearly those three stars stand in place of a name, and it seems to have been universally assumed that the name in place of which they stand is that of the author of the *Letter*. So with the secret of his identity now revealed, the name 'Diderot' can simply replace the three asterisks. Is this substitution legitimate?

Certainly the *Letter* tempts the reader to make the substitution. It contains, for example, a number of references to Condillac, the author of a number of important works of epistemological and linguistic theory, and Diderot was a friend of Condillac in this period.[18] Also, that part of the *Letter* which contains Saunderson's deathbed conversation is said in the text to be a translation from English,[19] and Diderot had been earning his living as a translator since 1743. He co-translated, for example, James's

---

14 Denis Diderot, *Lettre sur les aveugles*, Robert Niklaus (ed.) (Geneva: Droz, 1951), p. x.

15 Denis Diderot, *Œuvres philosophiques*, Paul Vernière (ed.) (Paris: Garnier, 1956), p. 8.

16 Diderot, DPV, vol. 4, p. 3. See also Colas Duflo, *Diderot philosophe* (Paris, Champion, 2003), p. 82.

17 Hobson and Harvey, p. 67; *Letter*, p. 219.

18 According to Rousseau, who said it was he who first introduced them, Diderot persuaded his own publisher, Durand, to take Condillac's first work, *Essai sur l'origine des connaissances humaines* [Essay on the Origin of Human Knowledge] (1746). Jean-Jacques Rousseau, *Confessions*, *Œuvres complètes*, Bernard Gagnebin and Marcel Raymond (eds), 5 volumes (Paris: Gallimard, 1959–1997), vol. 1, p. 347; *Confessions*, Angela Scholar (trans.) Patrick Coleman (ed., intro. and notes) (Oxford: Oxford World's Classics, 2008), pp. 337–8.

19 See Hobson and Harvey, p. 64; *Letter*, p. 203.

three-volume medical dictionary (1743–45) which appeared between 1746 and 1748 with the title *Dictionnaire universel de médecine*,[20] and translated Shaftesbury's *Essay on Virtue or Merit* (1699) which appeared in 1745 as *Essai sur le mérite et la vertu*.[21]

In spite of these and other details, however, which might encourage a conflation of the author and the first-person letter-writer, it is important to note that the *Letter* is not a real piece of Diderot's private correspondence that he has made public – it is not, for example, included in Georges Roth's edition of the correspondence, and nor should it be.[22] It is a fictional text in the epistolary genre. Moreover, one of the questions that the *Letter* raises is that of the distinction between fact and fiction, notably, as we'll see, in relation to 'the man-born-blind of Puiseaux' and the first-person narrative account of the visit to his house. A contradiction comes into view here for, given that readers have assumed the man-born-blind of Puiseaux to be an imaginary character, they must also implicitly have assumed the man who went to visit him to be imaginary too, yet they have referred to that visitor as 'Diderot'.[23] As we'll see, the man-born-blind turns out to be far from imaginary, but 'je' [I] is not necessarily Diderot, and given the interest exhibited in the work in blurring the lines between fact and fiction, it is particularly important to distinguish between the author of the *Letter* and the writer of the letter.

This, of course, begs the question of how to refer to the writer of the letter. For descriptive purposes, the 'letter-writer' is cumbersome, and the 'epistler' overly ecclesiastical, Pauline. The 'correspondent' is acceptable and will on occasion be used here, but the question is not simply one of description; it is also one of naming. It would be too longwinded to call him 'Your most humble and most obedient servant'; 'Asterisks' has too much phonetic interference from Goscinny and Uderzo's Gaulish rebel. Though readers of the Michelin Guide would no doubt be pleased to see the three asterisks translated into 'Vaut le Voyage' [Worth the Trip], given what we'll see is his digressive style, the two-star 'Vaut le Détour' [Worth the Detour] would be more appropriate. Anyway, there is something overly aristocratic about a composite name when the letter is not signed 'M. de ***' as many works of the period are, but simply '***'. Moreover, though three little stars were the standard way of signalling an ellipsis in eighteenth-century printing, that they appear in a work on blindness and

---

20 His co-translators were Eidous and Toussaint.

21 We should note how Diderot's title reverses the order of the nouns and alters the conjunction from 'or' to 'and'. As we'll see, the *Letter* abounds in internal reversals and tweaks of this kind.

22 See (or rather do not see) Denis Diderot, *Correspondence*, Georges Roth and Jean Varloot (eds), 16 volumes (Paris: Minuit, 1955–70).

23 I should know; I have done so myself.

therefore, to some extent, darkness is perhaps not insignificant. And so, though it may try the reader's patience and perhaps risk her eyesight, I have decided simply to call him what he calls himself, namely, ***.[24] How one might decide verbally to pronounce '***', I leave up to the reader, as does the author of the *Letter*.

There is another substitution or, at least, identification at work in many of the readings that claim that Diderot expresses his own atheist materialist point of view in the *Letter*. They rely on identifying Diderot with another character in the text: Saunderson, whose atheist materialist account of the origins of the universe, put forward on his deathbed, is given great prominence in the *Letter*.[25] Saunderson's account is certainly extremely striking both in its form – that of a reported dialogue with long passages of direct speech – and in its content, which is Epicurean, echoing Lucretius's *De Rerum Natura* in a manner not dissimilar to the emerging (though often clandestinely published) discourses of natural history such as Lamy's *De Principiis rerum* [On the Principles of Things] (1669), Maillet's *Telliamed* (c. 1692–1708, publ. 1748), Maupertuis's *Vénus physique* [Venus Embodied] (1745), La Mettrie's *L'Homme machine* [Machine Man] (1748) and Buffon's *Histoire naturelle* [Natural History] (1749–1777). Saunderson's arguments reduce his vicar to silence, but that is not necessarily a reason to take him simply to be a mouthpiece for Diderot. Moreover, when Saunderson has a last-minute change of heart and dies begging for divine forgiveness (albeit from a rather particular kind of God), either the identification of him as the voice of Diderot would seem to come unstuck or the claim that Diderot was by 1749 a confirmed atheist materialist would seem to require some modification. A further challenge to any conflation of *** with an atheist materialist Diderot is issued when the former expresses his approval of Saunderson's last words.

Those words and ***'s approval of them have often been overlooked by critics or swiftly dismissed as ironic.[26] Certainly the *Letter* makes much use of irony. However, in order to grasp how that irony works and, more importantly, in order to analyse how the text as a whole functions, the temptation simply to collapse different identities into each other needs to be resisted. I shall therefore observe distinctions between Saunderson and

---

24 It is perhaps noteworthy in this regard that in the edition held in the John Rylands Library (Manchester, UK), the first letter of the first word, the first-person personal pronoun, appears inside an ornament in the shape of a (single) star (see Figure 1).

25 Jean-Claude Bourdin has at least made his working hypothesis clear by stating, 'A supposer que Saunderson soit le pseudonyme de Diderot [. . .]' [Supposing that Saunderson is Diderot's pseudonym {. . .}], *Diderot. Le matérialisme*, p. 37.

26 Colas Duflo is a notable exception; his explanation of Saunderson's last words tends, however, to resolve its contradictions rather than explore them (see *Diderot philosophe*, pp. 99–100).

Diderot, between *** and Saunderson, and between Diderot, the writer of the anonymous *Letter*, and ***, the signatory to the letter to Madame.

The presence of atheist and of materialist Epicurean ideas in the *Letter* is extremely important. They have been expertly studied elsewere and this essay is indebted to that body of scholarship.[27] I also give equal attention and weight to other parts of the text, however, including the story of the visit to Puiseaux, the discussions of how the blind think, of geometry and of Molyneux's Problem, which many intellectual historians, philosophers and Diderot scholars have tended to overlook because they are not so radical or, rather, not as manifestly so. Such attention allows the presence of a much wider range of philosophical positions to come into view – sceptical, rationalist, empiricist, deist, atheist, materialist and idealist – and it makes visible the wayward manner in which the text moves from one position to the next. It also suggests not so much a break between the *Letter* and Diderot's earlier work as numerous continuities, notably with the *Pensées Philosophiques* [Philosophical Thoughts] (1746), a refutation of Pascal, with the pornographic novel *Les Bijoux indiscrets* [The Indiscreet Jewels] (1748), and the *Mémoires sur différents sujets de mathématiques* (1748).

Wider Focus and Closer Up

There have been some attempts to resist the critical tendency to focus almost exclusively on Saunderson's speech. A notable example of this kind of work is Colas Duflo's *Diderot philosophe* (2003), which reads other parts of the text both for themselves and with a view to how they might relate to each other.[28] This essay is indebted to his study, but it does not share his concern to make the case for Diderot as a philosopher and, in particular, as an atheist materialist philosopher, so it can afford to pay greater attention to the presence of other points of view in the *Letter*. A number of these are indicated in Harvey and Hobson's edition which, while having much to say about Saunderson, also points in numerous other directions and suggests by way of a comparison with the later *Lettre sur les sourds et muets* [Letter on the Deaf and the Dumb] (1751), which is devoted to linguistic theory, that the *Letter on the Blind* is 'moins une

27 See Jacques Roger, *Les sciences de la vie au XVIIIe siècle* (Paris: A. Colin, 1963); *The Life Sciences in Eighteenth-Century French Thought*, Keith R. Benson (ed.), Robert Ellrich (trans.) (Stanford: Stanford University Press, 1993); Ilya Prigogine and Isabelle Stengers, *La nouvelle alliance: métamorphose de la science* (Paris: Gallimard, 1986); *Order out of Chaos: Man's New Dialogue with Nature* (London: Heinemann, 1984); Ann Thomson, *Bodies of Thought: Science, Religion, and the Soul in the Early Enlightenment* (Oxford: Oxford University Press, 2008); Paolo Quintili, *Matérialismes et Lumières: philosophies de la vie, autour de Diderot et de quelques autres, 1706–1789* (Paris: Champion, 2009).

28 Duflo, *Diderot philosophe*, pp. 79–151.

affirmation avec thèse et thèmes qu'un parcours à travers différentes positions et une réflexion critique sur certaines opinions des contemporains' [not so much an affirmation with a thesis and themes as a journey through different positions and a critical reflection on some contemporaries' opinions].[29] This essay follows up some of their suggestions, and it charts that journey in detail.

My attention is also focused in this essay on the ways in which the text moves and on the moments at which it changes direction sometimes quite unpredictably and in ways that are calculated to produce deliberately ambiguous results. That this is a defining feature of Diderot's later writing has been observed by a number of critics who have studied it in depth. Jean Starobinski and Marian Hobson have provided detailed analyses of many of the later texts, identifying the manner in which the arguments often deploy patterns of anecdotes and particular syntactic features, such as parataxis and chiasmus, and pairs and triads of terms that echo, half-echo or contradict each other.[30] The earliest of Diderot's texts to receive this kind of close attention is the *Lettre sur les sourds et muets*, to which Hobson devoted an important article in 1976.[31]

The *Lettre sur les sourds et muets* is also the earliest text studied in Walter E. Rex's *Diderot's Counterpoints* (1998), in which he identifies what he calls a 'dynamics of contrariety' in Diderot's writing, a constant shuttling back and forth between positions, usually but not always voiced by different characters in dialogue. He claims that it is 'formidably confusing . . . erratically changing topics, changing assumptions, rendering obscure what has just been made plain, undoing what has just been done.'[32] This essay suggests that the *Letter on the Blind* is not, as it were, much better.

To do this, I draw on the method employed by Starobinski, Hobson and Rex, which might be called close reading, and on a number of studies devoted to the *Letter* that it also extends and refines. In *Le Style de Diderot* [Diderot's Style] (1986), Georges Daniel has explored what he calls the *Letter*'s 'mécanisme logico-syntaxique' [logico-syntactical mechanism], identifying symmetrical pairings (isocolon) and reversals (chiasmus).[33] With respect to the arguments of the *Letter*, Andrew Curran's *Sublime*

---

29 Hobson and Harvey, p. 10.

30 Jean Starobinski, 'Sur l'emploi du chiasme dans *Le Neveu de Rameau*'. *Revue de métaphysique et de morale*, 89.2 (1984), 182–96; Marian Hobson, *Diderot and Rousseau: Networks of Enlightenment. Collected Essays by Marian Hobson*, Kate E. Tunstall and Caroline Warman (ed. trans. and intro.), *SVEC*, 2011: 4.

31 See Marian Hobson, 'Diderot's *Letter on the Deaf and the Dumb*: Language and Labyrinth', in *Diderot and Rousseau*, pp. 213–59.

32 Walter E. Rex, *Diderot's Counterpoints: The Dynamics of Contrariety in his Major Works*. *SVEC*, 1998: 363, p. 60.

33 Georges Daniel, *Le style de Diderot: légende et structure* (Geneva and Paris: Droz, 1986), pp. 319–24.

Disorder (2001) shows how the different and sometimes contradictory ways in which blindness functions in the text relates to the changing status of the concept of the monstrous in France during the first half of the eighteenth century.[34] And in a number of studies, Jean-Claude Bourdin has observed and sought to resolve some other terminological and conceptual peculiarities in the text, notably concerning abstract thought and idealism.[35] This essay takes a different view: I argue that there are many places in the *Letter* in which the writing is not so much symmetrical and binary as lopsided and off-balance, that the significance and paradoxes of blindness are not limited to the question of monstrosity, and that contradiction and ambiguity, terminological slips and flips are an important and deliberate feature of the text's dynamics which require observation and analysis rather than resolution and straightening out.

But why write like this? Rex offers a psychological explanation for the *Letter*'s shifts, swerves and contradictions, claiming they were 'unconscious, unexamined', and that Diderot 'remained deaf, dumb and blind to the essentials of his own thinking processes.'[36] This essay rejects a psychological explanation for the shifts and swerves of Diderot's writing. They may be unacknowledged by *** (though, in fact, that is far from always the case), but that is not at all the same thing as Diderot being 'unconscious' of them. I argue instead that the *Letter* engages in what we might think of as a number of deliberately destabilising interpretive games.

Blind Man's Buff

To some extent, the *Letter* exhibits the same sort of dynamic that is present in Montaigne's 'Apologie de Raimond Sebond' [Apology for Raimond Sebond], a text Diderot knew well.[37] Focusing on the nature of the writing in the essay rather than on the rather dead-end question of whether or not the author was a sceptic, Terence Cave's *Pré-histoires I* [Pre-Histories I] (1999) has identified the volte-face dynamic of antiperistasis. This involves the disconcerting conversion of a term into its opposite by, for instance, varying the rhythms of a sentence or subtly altering its frame of reference,

34 Andrew Curran, *Sublime Disorder: Physical Monstrosity in Diderot's Universe. SVEC*, 2001: 1, pp. 58–79. For a study of the early modern monster, see Wes Williams, *Monsters and their Meanings in Early Modern Culture. Mighty Magic* (Oxford: Oxford University Press, 2011).

35 Bourdin, *Diderot. Le matérialisme*, pp. 39–40; 'Le matérialisme dans la *Lettre sur les aveugles*'. *Recherches sur Diderot et l'Encyclopédie*, 28 (2000), 83–96.

36 Rex, 'Diderot's Counterpoints', p. 309.

37 See Schwartz, *Diderot and Montaigne*. Rex briefly compares Montaigne and Diderot, but he claims the comparison is unworkable because while Montaigne was conscious of his changeability, Diderot was not (*Diderot's Counterpoints*, p. 309). His main points of comparison are instead La Fontaine, Molière and Voltaire, (*Diderot's Counterpoints*, pp. 1–25).

only then to return it to its official meaning.[38] Such movements are also discernible in Diderot's later work.[39] In the *Letter*, terms such as 'blind' and 'abstract' undergo a change in value in a manner that is not dissimilar to the terminological 'transvaluations' that Cave identifies in the 'Apology'. Moreover, positions and rhythms we might identify with Montaigne are sometimes themselves made to function in the *Letter* as the official meaning.

If Montaigne is one writing model, *** explicitly suggests two others. He identifies two kinds of writing – one 'precious' and one 'obscure'.[40] The former is cryptically said to be that of 'M. de M . . .'. In the Index to the *Letter*, a paratext compiled by Diderot which supplies a number of clues to the text, the identity of 'M. de M . . .' is revealed to be the journalist, novelist and playwright, Marivaux. The literal back and forth movement involved in turning to the Index, discovering Marivaux's name and returning to the main text might itself be said to mime the to and fro dynamic of the 'precious' style associated with Marivaux, his preference for curves, swerves and loops over straight lines which characterises the 'rocaille' æsthetic, now usually referred to as 'rococo' (although that term did not appear until the nineteenth century).[41] Hobson and Harvey have alluded to the possibility that 'rocaille' might apply to both the *Letter on the Blind* and the *Lettre sur les sourds et muets*,[42] though Hobson has only explicitly made the argument with reference to the latter work.[43] In her article 'Philosophy and Rococo Style' (2002), she associates 'rocaille' with an æsthetic of disorder that she discerns in Diderot's writing from

38 Terence Cave, *Pré-histoires. Textes troublés au seuil de la modernité* (Geneva: Droz, 1999), p. 49. See also Cave, 'Imagining Scepticism in the Sixteenth Century', in *Retrospectives: Essays in Literature, Poetics and Cultural History*, Neil Kenny and Wes Williams (eds) (Oxford: Legenda, 2009), p. 126. Cave gives a psychological explanation for the way Montaigne writes, describing the 'Apologie' as a 'texte troublé' [troubled text] and defining textual trouble as a 'signe textuel d'une réponse psychologique à un phénomène qui pour nous est historique' [textual sign of a psychological response to a phenomenon that is historical for us], *Pré-histoires*, p. 16.

39 For a specific comparison between Montaigne and Diderot, see Schwartz, *Montaigne and Diderot*; and Kate E. Tunstall, 'Portraits and Afterlives: Diderot and Montaigne', in Anna Holland and Richard Scholar (eds), *Pre-Histories and Afterlives: Studies in Critical Method for Terence Cave* (London: Legenda, 2009), pp. 95–105.

40 Hobson and Harvey, p. 54; *Letter*, p. 194.

41 The OED gives the first English usage as 1830, and the first dictionary entry for the French term is to be found in Émile Littré, *Dictionnaire de la langue française* [Dictionary of the French Language] (Paris: Hachette, 1872–77).

42 They conclude their Presentation of the two *Letters* saying that they have 'un style rococo, pourrait-on dire' [a rococo style, one might say] (Hobson and Harvey, p. 24).

43 Hobson, 'Philosophy and Rococo Style' in *Diderot and Rousseau*, pp. 203–12.

1751 onwards, though she argues that it owes something to the concept of nature as disordered that was first articulated in the earlier letter by Saunderson.[44] My essay takes the opportunity offered by the references to Marivaux and preciosity in the *Letter*, which Hobson overlooks, to develop and nuance her claim, linking the *Letter* to 'rocaille' not so much because it is a disordered æsthetic as because it offers variations on the theme of sight that involve reflections, reversals and refractions. It is not for nothing that the *Letter on the Blind* includes a discussion of mirrors.

This complex dynamic, which we might think of as a kind of 'radical rococo', is deliberately designed not only, as any literary text in the long sceptical tradition might be said to, to refuse a single point of view or, rather, to show up 'point of view' as 'point de vue' – the French term means both 'point of view' and 'no view at all'; it is also calculated constantly to shift the grounds on which philosophical enquiry can proceed, let alone receive any reliable answers. ***'s praise for Condillac's *Traité des systèmes* [Treatise on Systems] (1749) is important in this regard: the work is a critique of systems of thought, of system-thinking. Although, on one occasion, *** accuses Condillac of having succumbed to a system himself, it would be difficult, perhaps impossible, to level such an accusation at the *Letter*.

The 'obscure' kind of writing is said, straightforwardly, to be that of Tacitus. The reference to the Roman historian is also important for my study. His Latin is indeed obscure; it is both deeply ironic and syntactically elliptical.[45] In later works by Diderot, Tacitus is said to be 'toujours obscur par sa briéveté et son sens profond' [always obscure owing to his brevity and buried meaning],[46] 'le Rembrandt de la littérature: des ombres fortes, et des clairs éblouissants.' [the Rembrandt of literature: dark shadows and dazzling lights].[47] Many historians have argued that Tacitus' style is a function of the content and context of his writing, which denounced the tyranny of an Empire that prohibited freedom of speech.[48]

---

44 Hobson, *Diderot and Rousseau*, pp. 207–10.

45 In the early 1740s, Rousseau remarked: 'j'ai de l'aversion pour Tacite dont on ne perce l'obscurité qu'avec des peines qui sont souvent à pure perte pour les lecteurs. Je ne puis souffrir ce raffinement outré ni cette manière pointilleuse de chercher à tout des motifs subtils et mystérieux.' [I have an aversion to Tacitus whose veil of obscurity can only be pierced with great effort, which often brings readers no reward. I cannot bear that excessive refinement nor that pernickety way he has of seeking subtle and mysterious motives behind everything.] *Mémoire à M. de Mably* (1740–43) (quoted in Catherine Volpilhac-Auger, *Tacite en France de Montesquieu à Chateaubriand. SVEC*, 313 (1993), p. 4).

46 Quoted in Volpilhac-Auger, *Tacite en France*, p. 523.

47 Quoted in Volpilhac-Auger, *Tacite en France*, p. 523, note 26.

48 See, for example, Ellen O'Gorman, *Irony and Misreading in the Annals of Tacitus* (Cambridge: Cambridge University Press, 2000), pp. 1–14.

In light of this, the explicit reference to Tacitus in the *Letter*, as well as to particular kinds of reader, described as 'certaines gens qui voient du crime à tout' [some people who see crime everywhere], might be read as an encouragement to take the text's dynamic asymmetries and arresting formulations as games with the censor.

Of course, it might also be said that the *Letter* took its games too far or, rather, that the evidence for the text as playful is rather shaky, since Diderot was arrested in late July 1749, two months after the publication of the *Letter*.[49] It is important, however, to resist reading the *Letter* in a proleptic light and to guard against conflating the real police, who would later arrest Diderot, with what we might instead think of as a kind of imaginary thought-police invented by *** in the *Letter* for his own purposes. Hindsight blinds us to the text's ironies, tempts us into resolving its ambiguities and thereby obstructs or, at least, seriously impoverishes our reading. Moreover, if *** refers to the 'people who see crime everywhere' and who make him darken the clarity of his writing, it is because they are an integral part of the game of nods and winks that *** is playing with Madame: it is they who both authorize his transgressions and guarantee that we read them as such.

The *Letter* engages us then in a game of interpretive hide-and-seek or, more appropriately (not least because it is a topos of rococo painting),[50] blind man's buff. Sometimes we are the blindfolded figure who is spun around by the text as positions flip, terminology slips and we lose our footing; at other times, the reader joins in with *** to spin the censor round, sneak behind his back, avoid his clutches and enjoy getting caught. An early version of this game can be found in the *Letter*'s epigraph.

The Epigraph

The epigraph has escaped detailed critical commentary to date, but it sets the tone for some of the ironies and ambiguities to be found in the text that bears it on its title page. It reads, '*Possunt,* nec *posse videntur*'. Attributed to Virgil, it is adapted from Book Five, line 231 of the *Æneid*, which reads 'Possunt, quia posse videntur'. Depending on whether 'videntur' is taken to be reflexive or not, the line means either 'They can, because they think they can' or 'They can because they are seen to be able to'.[51] In the first instance, Virgil's phrase is a paean to the power of positive thinking; in

49 For a detailed account of his arrest that reproduces many of the police documents, see Paul Bonnefon, 'Diderot à Vincennes'. *Revue de l'Histoire Littéraire de la France*, 6 (1899), 200–24.

50 For a study of the five paintings on this theme by Jean-Honoré Fragonard, see Jennifer Milam, 'Fragonard and the Blindman's Game'. *Art History*, 21.1 (1998), 1–25.

51 Hobson and Harvey, p. 173, note 1.

the second, it makes a claim for causal links between seeing, seeming and power.[52] The *Letter*'s epigraph replaces Virgil's causal relationship, 'quia', with an opposition, 'nec': 'They can, *though* they don't look as though they can'.[53] On the one hand, having no eyes but being able nonetheless to see could easily sound miraculous, and one contemporary reader (to whom we shall return) says that the epigraph 'fait allusion aux prodiges des aveugles-nés.' [alludes to the wonders of men-born-blind.][54] On the other hand, it announces the redundancy of the cataract operation since men-born-blind can see already. And so it also subtly suggests the redundancy of the Christian revelation – the blind unbeliever is clear-sighted in his unbelief.[55]

The epigraph also sets up a fundamental contrast between appearance and reality. Its claim is not simply that the blind can see; it is also that the blind are *trompe l'œil* – they don't look as though they can see, but they can. The contrast is binary but there are three points of view available here: that of the sighted (to whom it seems that the blind cannot see), that of the blind (to whom, depending on whether 'videntur' is read as reflexive or not, it may also seem that they cannot see), and that of the epigrapher (who is not deceived). But who is the latter? Is he sighted or blind? Does he know the blind can see because he is blind too? Does he have the confidence of the blind, which he is about to break by divulging their secret in the *Letter*? If so, he might be akin to the hero of Diderot's earlier pornographic novel, *Les Bijoux indiscrets*, who impertinently reveals women's hidden desires by making their genitalia speak. Or is he a kind of mega-seer who can see through appearances and see what no one else can and know what even the blind themselves do not know, namely that they have the power of sight? If so, he might be akin to the cataract surgeon who makes the blind see and enlightens the sighted.

By way of its reference to appearances that are deceptive, the epigraph also evokes the mottoes that appeared in or on many anonymous libertine works and which refer to masking, hiding and other acts of

---

52 See Andrew Feldherr, 'Ships of State: *Aeneid* 5 and Augustan Circus Spectacle'. *Classical Antiquity*, 14.2 (1995), 245–65, 259.

53 The alteration is signalled typographically – 'nec' is the only word not in italics.

54 'Aveugle' [Blind Man], in *Encyclopédie, ou Dictionnaire raisonné des sciences, des arts et des métiers*, 28 volumes (Paris: Le Breton, Briasson, David and Durand, 1751–72), vol. 1, p. 870.

55 The epigraph echoes and inverts numerous lines in the Bible, see Romans 11.8; Mark 8.18; John 9.25 and 12.40.

dissimulation.[56] It thereby suggests that the text may itself be *trompe l'œil* too; if the reader is to see, she may have to pierce some kind of veil. This also introduces a third figure into the relationship between writer and reader, between *** and Madame, namely the censor, whose eyes are to be tricked by the text. Blind man's buff starts even before the *Letter* has begun.

In order to ensure my reader does not feel herself blindfolded and unexpectedly spun round, a brief guide to the essay may be of use. Overall, my approach is two-fold. It proceeds by means of a close reading of the *Letter*, paying particular attention to intertextual echoes that locate the text in a larger philosophical and literary tradition. Given this attention to echoes, the 'close' in my close reading is not only visual; it is also and, perhaps to a greater degree, aural. In addition, the approach involves accepting an invitation that, I argue, the *Letter* issues to the reader – namely, to take part in a conversation.[57] By reading the *Letter* with an eye and an ear to its literary features, I show that it requires the reader to supply for herself certain ideas and words at which it only hints, though it sometimes draws attention to the hint. To some degree, then, my essay is speculative, responding to aural and visual cues and clues in the *Letter*, and sharing in the production of the text's meanings and the formulation of its questions.

Six chapters follow this Introduction. The first, 'Reading is Believing?', explores the *Letter*'s original response to the widespread interest in blindness in the period, generated by Molyneux's Problem, which is to go in search of real men-born-blind. The chapter provides the results of some detective work which shows that the men-born-blind of the *Letter* are complex combinations of fact and fiction, and it focuses on the ways in which the text draws attention to their status as such, arguing that this is designed to set the reader on her guard both against believing what she reads and dismissing it as made up.

In telling stories of men-born-blind, the *Letter* is an heir to a tradition, and this is explored in the second chapter, 'The Blind Leading the Blind Leading the Blind Leading the Blind Leading the Blind . . .'. In it,

56 We might think of 'bene vixit qui bene latuit' [he who lives hidden, lives well], taken from Ovid's *Tristia*, 3: 4, line 25, or Descartes's 'Larvatus prodeo' [Masked, I go forth]. For analyses of libertine writing strategies, see Jean-Pierre Cavaillé, *Dissimulations. Religion, morale et politique au XVIIe siècle* (Paris: Champion, 2002). Bourdin disagrees that the libertine tradition of dissimulation is relevant to the *Letter* ('Le matérialisme dans la *Lettre sur les aveugles*', p. 86).

57 For a study of the importance of conversation to Enlightenment modes of intellectual exchange, see Lawrence Klein, 'Enlightenment as Conversation' in Keith Baker and Peter Reill (eds), *What's Left of Enlightenment? A Postmodern Question* (Stanford: Stanford University Press, 2001), pp. 148–66.

I explore the men-born-blind of sceptical, freethinking, Cartesian and anti-Cartesian writing, as well as the blind men of pre-modern and early modern farce.

Such texts often present men-born-blind not merely as silent signs to be deciphered by their sighted observers, but as men with their own perspectives on the world and their own stories to tell, and so in the third chapter, 'Point of View and *Point de Vue*', I analyse the *Letter*'s narrative of the visit to see the man-born-blind of Puiseaux and hear what he has to say, particularly on the subjects of morals and metaphysics. The chapter pays particular attention to the way the text presents both the point of view of the man-born-blind of Puiseaux and the effect that observing and listening to him has on ***'s own point of view. It shows that the *Letter* exploits the duality that the French phrase 'point de vue' makes so felicitously audible: meaning both 'point of view' and 'no view at all', it suggests that every point of view is also a blind alley.

A fairly abrupt shift in the *Letter* away from anecdotal narrative to discursive speculation triggers a new chapter in this essay. Chapter Four, 'Groping Around in the Light', attends to the exploration of the sense of touch and its seemingly contradictory associations with both the material body and abstract thought, which I suggest links the *Letter* to both Descartes and Berkeley as well as to the anti-Cartesian art theory of Roger de Piles. It is in this chapter that I also consider the practice of allusion in the *Letter* and its theory as presented in the series of remarks about the particular ways in which the blind and other outsiders, such as foreigners and talented writers, use language.

If Saunderson's deathbed is the most well-known part of the *Letter*, it is no doubt because Saunderson expresses his views in a manner that is, by contrast, far from allusive; instead it is extremely direct, and those views and their presentation are the subject of the fifth chapter, 'A Supplement to Saunderson's "Memoirs"'. In addition to providing a gloss on Saunderson's scepticism with regard to the existence of God, and his alternative, Epicurean account of the origins of the universe, the chapter considers his very last words and ***'s commentary on them, suggesting links to works by Bayle, La Mettrie and Pascal, as well as to the 'Memoirs' of the real Saunderson. What emerges here is a complex picture of the way in which Saunderson's views are presented in the *Letter* and one that unexpectedly lays the ground for the original treatment of Molyneux's Problem in the final section of the text.

'Dis/Solving Molyneux's Problem' is my final chapter, which explains the *Letter*'s answer to Molyneux's epistemological brainteaser and, more importantly, shows how it goes far beyond any contemporaneous discussion owing to its consideration of the question of the body in pain. I show how the *Letter* contrasts the physical pain involved in the cataract surgery, which may also be pointlessly painful if the blind can see anyway, with the metaphysical pain felt by Saunderson, who experiences his blindness as a deprivation that seems to have been gratuitously inflicted since he was born blind. There are theological implications here that have not been observed before.

The aim of the essay, then, is not so much to answer the questions raised in and by the *Letter* as to reveal how the text goes about raising the questions it does and, perhaps most importantly, to preserve its complex, interrogative nature. My hope is that, having read the essay, the reader will be prepared for reading or re-reading Diderot's *Letter* (either in the French original or in the new translation that can be found here in the Appendix), and for taking up its invitation to participate in a conversation of the most enlightening and enlivening kind.

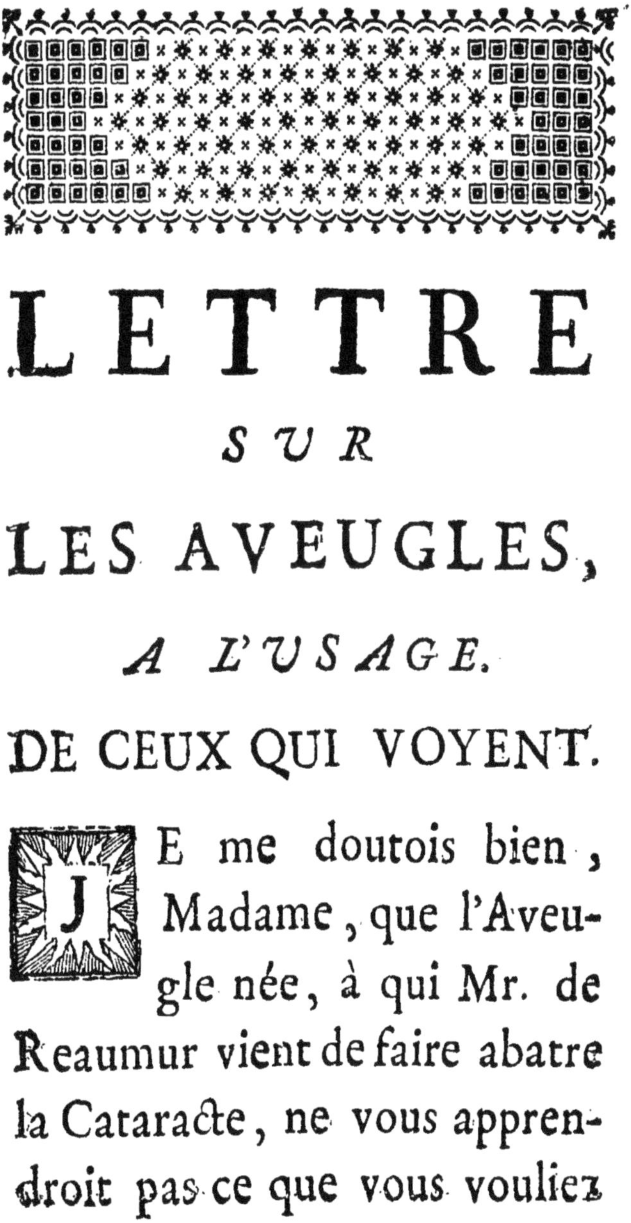

LETTRE

SUR

LES AVEUGLES,

A L'USAGE.

DE CEUX QUI VOYENT.

JE me doutois bien, Madame, que l'Aveugle née, à qui Mr. de Reaumur vient de faire abatre la Cataracte, ne vous apprendroit pas ce que vous vouliez

Figure 1 First page of *Lettre sur les aveugles* (London [Paris], 1749). Reproduced courtesy of the University Librarian and Director, The John Rylands Library, The University of Manchester.

One

Reading is Believing?

The opening paragraph of the *Letter* is sufficiently complex to merit being quoted here in full. It stages a scene, which involves not a mother and a son, but two women, both awaiting enlightenment. It goes like this:

> Je me doutais bien, Madame, que l'aveugle-née, à qui M. de Réaumur vient de faire abattre la cataracte, ne nous apprendrait pas ce que vous vouliez savoir; mais je n'avais garde de deviner que ce ne serait ni sa faute, ni la vôtre. J'ai sollicité son bienfaiteur par moi-même, par ses meilleurs amis, par les compliments que je lui ai faits; nous n'en avons rien obtenu, et le premier appareil se lèvera sans vous. Des personnes de la première distinction ont eu l'honneur de partager son refus avec les philosophes; en un mot, il n'a voulu laisser tomber le voile que devant quelques yeux sans conséquence. Si vous êtes curieuse de savoir pourquoi cet habile académicien fait si secrètement des expériences qui ne peuvent avoir, selon vous, un trop grand nombre de témoins éclairés, je vous répondrai que les observations d'un homme aussi célèbre ont moins besoin de spectateurs, quand elles se font, que d'auditeurs, quand elles sont faites. Je suis donc revenu, Madame, à mon premier dessein; et forcé de me passer d'une expérience où je ne voyais guère à gagner pour mon instruction ni pour la vôtre, mais dont M. de Réaumur tirera sans doute un bien meilleur parti, je me suis mis à philosopher avec mes amis sur la matière importante qu'elle a pour objet. Que je serais heureux, si le récit d'un de nos entretiens pouvait me tenir lieu auprès de vous du spectacle que je vous avais trop légèrement promis![1]

> I had my doubts, Madame, about whether the blind girl whose cataracts Monsieur de Réaumur has just had removed, would reveal to you what you wanted to know, but it had not occurred to me that it would be neither her fault nor yours. I have appealed

1 DPV, 4, p. 17; Hobson and Harvey, p. 29.

> to her benefactor in person and through his best friends, as well as by means of flattery, but to no avail, and the first dressing will be removed without you. Some highly distinguished people have shared with the philosophers the honour of being snubbed by him. In a word, he only wanted to perform the unveiling in front of eyes of no consequence. Should you be curious to know why that talented Academician makes such a secret of his experiments, which cannot, in your view, have too great a number of enlightened witnesses, I should reply that the observations of such a famous man do not so much need spectators while they are being performed as an audience once the performance is over. So, Madame, I have returned to my initial plan, and having no choice but to miss out on an experiment which I could not see would be instructive for either you or me, but which will doubtless serve Monsieur de Réaumur rather better, I began philosophizing with my friends on the important matter that it concerns. How delighted I should be were you to accept the account of one of our conversations as a substitute for the spectacle that I so rashly promised you![2]

So Madame is to be disappointed. Not because the girl's operation has failed nor because she has herself been inattentive, but rather because she will not be allowed to see the spectacle. *** has failed to obtain permission for Madame and himself to witness the dressing coming off. And it's not for want of trying, as he is at pains to point out; Réaumur – the eminent scientist, sometime Director of the Académie Royale des Sciences and, perhaps most significantly, microscopist – has deliberately blocked their view.[3] He is presented here as hostile to the philosophers, with whom *** says he and Madame have had the honour of sharing his snub, and as vain, far more concerned with his own reputation than with the public dissemination of scientific knowledge. So the girl-born-blind will get her sight or, rather, others will see whether she will be able to see (that is, whether she will be able to recognize objects that were familiar to her touch), but *** and Madame will be left in the dark.

However, while *** makes it clear that it was the myopic Réaumur's preference for marvellous tales of his own great works that was responsible for their being unable to witness the revelation, he does not present access to empirical, visual evidence as most important, nor does he set up a stable opposition between seeing and hearing in which the former is preferable to the latter. Far from it, in fact; though Réaumur's preference for hearing is satirized, it turns out to be the sense that *** also prefers,

2 *Letter*, p. 171.

3 For a biography, see Jean Torlais, *Réaumur: un esprit encyclopédique en dehors de l'Encyclopédie* (Paris: Librairie Blanchard, 1961).

calling into question the merits of vision and visual spectacle as he tells Madame that he never thought the unveiling was going to be enlightening and at first had it in mind to converse with his friends about the 'important matter that it concerns', an allusion to Molyneux's Problem. So Réaumur is presented as having unwittingly proved *** right, and moreover, a blocked view is no obstacle; indeed it facilitates ***'s 'initial plan'. Moreover that plan, a conversation with friends, is now one in which Madame can be included.

So, while Madame's expectations may have been dashed by Réaumur's preference for self-serving myths, Réaumur's decision to keep her and *** in the dark has provided the latter with the perfect opportunity to indulge his preference for storytelling and conversation over visual spectacle and empirical evidence. And so, the letter that *** has sent to Madame will not so much involve recognition or misrecognition scenes as a conversation and tales of conversations about and with men-born-blind who stay blind but can nonetheless or, rather, for precisely that reason, enlighten the sighted. Let's meet them.

The Man-Born-Blind of Puiseaux

Before we do so, it is important to note that some of the difficulties observed earlier with respect to identifying *** with the historical person, Diderot, and the censorious reader with the historical censor, also surround both the men-born-blind of the *Letter*. Both are presented in ways that raise tricky questions about their status as fact or fiction. In the first section of the *Letter*, *** tells Madame about the visit that he and his friends made to the home of the man-born-blind of Puiseaux. This is a figure to whom critics have not paid much attention or, at least, not nearly as much as they have to Saunderson,[4] and yet not only does he richly repay our attention, but *** explicitly asks Madame to make a judgement about his status as real or imaginary.

The manner in which he is introduced to Madame is worth quoting in full:

> Le jour même que le Prussien faisait l'opération de la cataracte à la fille de Simoneau, nous allâmes interroger l'aveugle-né du Puiseaux*: c'est un homme qui ne manque pas de bon sens; que beaucoup de personnes connaissent; qui sait un peu de chimie, et qui a suivi, avec quelques succès, les cours de botanique au Jardin du Roi. Il est né d'un père qui a professé avec applaudissement la philosophie dans l'université de Paris. Il jouissait d'une fortune honnête, avec laquelle il eût aisément satisfait les sens qui lui restent;

4 An exception is Markovits, 'Mérian, Diderot et l'aveugle', pp. 193–282.

mais le goût du plaisir l'entraîna dans sa jeunesse: on abusa de ses penchants; ses affaires domestiques se dérangèrent, et il s'est retiré dans une petite ville de province, d'où il fait tous les ans un voyage à Paris. Il y apporte des liqueurs qu'il distille, et dont on est très content. Voilà, Madame, des circonstances assez peu philosophiques, mais par cette raison même, plus propres à vous faire juger, que le personnage dont je vous entretiens n'est point imaginaire.

* Petite ville du Gâtinais.[5]

The very day that the Prussian was performing the cataract operation on Simoneau's daughter, we went to question the man-born-blind of Puiseaux.* He is a man not lacking in good sense, with whom many people are acquainted, who knows a bit of chemistry and followed the botany lessons quite successfully in the King's Garden. His father taught philosophy to much acclaim in the University of Paris and left him an honest fortune, which would easily have been enough to satisfy his remaining senses, had his love of pleasure not led him astray in his youth. People took advantage of his inclinations, and he retired to a little town in the provinces whence he comes to Paris once a year, bringing with him liqueurs of his own distillation, which are much appreciated. There you have some details, Madame, which, though not very philosophical, are for that very reason all the more suitable for persuading you that the character of whom I am speaking is not imaginary.

* Small town in the Gâtinais.[6]

So while a girl-born-blind, perhaps the daughter of one of the engravers of Réaumur's *Mémoires pour servir à l'histoire des insectes* [Memoirs for Use in the History of Insects] (1734–42),[7] was being operated on by the Prussian surgeon, Josef Hillmer,[8] *** and his friends went off to Puiseaux to ask some questions of a man-born-blind. While Mademoiselle Simoneau was being made to see, the man-born-blind of Puiseaux was being made to speak.

*** had rather allusively cast some doubts as to Mademoiselle Simoneau's suitability for the experiment when he said he had thought

5 DPV, 4, p. 18; Hobson and Harvey, p. 29–30.
6 *Letter*, pp. 171–2.
7 René Antoine Ferchault, seigneur de Réaumur et de La Bermondière, *Mémoires pour servir à l'histoire des insectes*, 6 volumes (Paris: Imprimerie Royale, 1734–42). The four engravers were Simoneau, Lucas, Haussard and Fillioeul.
8 We will return to him later, see below, pp. 127–30.

she might be responsible for Réaumur's experiment not being a success. He will not fully explain what he means until much later in the *Letter*, but a clue is offered here in the details of the man-born-blind-of-Puiseaux's background and various accomplishments, all of which implicitly contrast him with what we assume to be those of an engraver's daughter. They suggest that, though blind, he might be able to enlighten Madame. Moreover, he received some of his education at the Académie's rival institution, the 'Jardin du Roi' [King's Garden] which, as Emma Spary has shown in *Utopia's Garden* (2000), was identified with its Director, Buffon, whose aim since his appointment in 1739 had been to obtain a place for the Jardin du Roi within the political and cultural economy akin to that of the Académie royale des sciences with which Réaumur was identified.[9] And, as has often been remarked, the differences between Réaumur and Buffon were also philosophical: the account of the natural world given by the former in a work such as the *Mémoires pour servir à l'histoire des insectes* was resolutely deist – seen under the microscope, even the tiniest of insects revealed a design that proclaimed the existence of a divine designer, whereas that offered by the latter's *Histoire naturelle* [Natural History] (1749–1788) found little place for a divine plan.[10] Already the first two paragraphs of the *Letter*, containing an overt and hostile reference to Réaumur and a covert and implicitly positive reference to Buffon, are suggestive of the sympathies of the text that follows.

If the man-born-blind-of-Puiseaux's reliability is thus established and his allegiances suggested, *** nonetheless raises a question as to his own reliability: 'Voilà, Madame, des circonstances assez peu philosophiques, mais par cette raison même, plus propres à vous faire juger, que le personnage dont je vous entretiens n'est point imaginaire' [There you have some details, Madame, which, though not very philosophical, are for that very reason all the more suitable for persuading you that the character of whom I am speaking is not imaginary].[11] Moreover, such 'not very philosophical' details are strengthened in the footnote containing information as to the precise geographical whereabouts of the town of Puiseaux.[12] What are we to make of the fact that *** draws our attention to his attempt to persuade Madame that the man-born-blind of Puiseaux is a real person, or rather, a 'not imaginary' one, and how are we to judge

9 Emma Spary, *Utopia's Garden: French Natural History from Old Regime to Revolution* (Chicago: Chicago University Press, 2000).

10 G. L. Leclerc, comte de Buffon, *Histoire naturelle, générale et particulière, avec la description du cabinet du roy*, 36 volumes (Paris: Imprimerie royale, 1749–88).

11 DPV, 4, p. 18; Hobson and Harvey, p. 30.

12 Many editors supplement the existing footnote with another, explaining in further geographical detail where Puiseaux is located; see DPV, 4, p. 18, note 7; Hobson and Harvey, p. 129.

him: fact or fiction?

Critical opinion is divided as to whether or not *** is insinuating that the man-born-blind of Puiseaux is imaginary. Andrew Curran has remarked on the 'detached journalistic manner' in which the man-born-blind of Puiseaux is presented, suggesting he takes him to be real, but he omits the final reflexive remark to Madame, presumably for its rather non-journalistic manner.[13] Colas Duflo, by contrast, is of the view not only that the man-born-blind of Puiseaux is imaginary, but also that Diderot is alerting us to this fact in the final remark to Madame (whom he takes to be fictional also), which is the only part of the paragraph that he quotes.[14] Marian Hobson and Simon Harvey's edition of the *Letter* hedges its bets, observing that the remark to Madame is typical of novels of the period and also noting that in a work entitled *The Story of Blindness* (1956), Gabriel Farrell has stated that the man-born-blind-of-Puiseaux's name was 'Lenôtre'.[15]

A closer examination of Farrell's claim reveals that it should be dismissed. It is based on a simple misunderstanding of the possessive pronoun in French: *** often refers to the man-born-blind of Puiseaux as 'notre aveugle' [our blind man] and also, on occasion, as 'le nôtre' [ours]. Wrong though it is, Farrell's claim highlights the frequent use of the possessive pronoun in the *Letter*, a feature to which we shall return. Yet if Hobson and Harvey were motivated to report Farrell's claim by some sense that the man-born-blind of Puiseaux might not be imaginary, they were right. *** is not the unreliable narrator Duflo has taken him to be or, at least, not quite. And the real-life existence of 'our' blind man points to new links between the *Letter on the Blind* and the *Encyclopédie*, which both authorize some degree of connection between *** and Diderot and introduce us to another starry persona, namely, *.

The Encyclopédie: Blind Men and Bonnets

In 1747, Diderot signed a contract that was the most important of his life: the co-editorship with d'Alembert of the *Encyclopédie*. It was secured to a great extent on the basis of his work as a translator since the *Encyclopédie* was originally conceived as a translation of Chambers's *Cyclopædia*, but the *Pensées philosophiques* is likely to have contributed also: it had been condemned by the Parlement as contrary to religion and moral decency and, as a result, it enjoyed a certain 'succès de scandale'.[16] The publisher of the *Pensées* was Laurent Durand, who would later distribute the *Letter*

13 Curran, *Sublime Disorder*, p. 77.
14 Duflo, *Diderot philosophe*, p. 87.
15 Hobson and Harvey, p. 173, note 8.
16 See Robert Morin, *Les Pensées philosophiques de Diderot devant leurs principaux contradicteurs au XVIIIe siècle* (Paris: Belles Lettres, 1975).

(and following its commercial success, publish other editions later in 1749), and he was also one of the four associated printers and booksellers for the *Encyclopédie*.[17] When they engaged Diderot as co-editor, they were no doubt in part also seeking further success of a kind similar to that of the *Pensées*. They would not be disappointed.

By mid 1749, work on the *Encyclopédie* was well underway[18] and the first volume, containing articles from 'A' to 'Azymites', appeared in June 1751. That first volume also contains 'Aveugle' [Blind Man] and 'Aveugles' [Blind Men] – articles that reveal the two co-editors behaving in particularly playful ways. The first article, 'Blind Man', is signed by '0'; the second, 'Blind Men', by '*'. A key, provided in the 'Avertissement' [Notice],[19] tells us that '0' is d'Alembert – perhaps because his full name was Jean Le Rond [The Circle] d'Alembert, and '*' is Diderot. We don't know what motivated Diderot's choice of symbol, but a single star was the standard mark for a footnote, and so it might be that, as an editor, he figured himself as a kind of footnote to the work of other people, a position that is not quite as self-effacing as it might sound in an era when footnotes could be, as they were in Bayle's dictionary, much longer and far more interesting than the rest of the text.[20] If this were right, it would be possible to suggest a link between the asterisk indicating the footnote supplying geographical information as to the location of Puiseaux in the *Letter* and *, since *-Diderot also provided many of the articles on geography in the first volumes of the *Encyclopédie*.

In 'Aveugle', 0 gives a somewhat expurgated summary of a recent anonymous publication, entitled the *Letter on the Blind*.[21] It is expurgated no doubt because by the time the first volume appeared, Diderot had been arrested and then released, largely, it would seem, thanks to the petitions sent to various members of the government by the printers and booksellers involved in the *Encyclopédie*, who stood to lose a small fortune if one of their editors remained in detention for long. 0, * and the *libraires* would have been keen to try and ensure that nothing like it happened again. Indeed, there are occasions on which 0 suggests a more orthodox

17 The other printers and booksellers were Briasson, David l'aîné and Le Breton.

18 For histories of the *Encyclopédie*, see Jacques Proust, *Diderot et l'Encyclopédie* (Paris: Albin Michel, 1962); John Lough, *Essays on the Encyclopédie of Diderot and D'Alembert* (London: Oxford University Press, 1968); Robert Darnton, *The Business of Enlightenment: a Publishing History of the Encyclopédie, 1775–1800* (Cambridge, Mass: Bellknap Publishing, 1979); and the numerous articles in the journal *Recherches sur Diderot et l'Encyclopédie*.

19 *Encyclopédie*, vol. 1, p. xlvi.

20 Given the importance accorded to artisans in the *Encyclopédie*, * could also be a kind of maker's mark, recalling those used by artisans to sign to their work. I am grateful to Katie Scott for this suggestion.

21 'Aveugle', in *Encyclopédie*, vol. 1, p. 870–3.

reading of the *Letter* in his article: he is the contemporary reader to whom we referred earlier, who claimed the epigraph made reference to the 'prodiges' [wonders] of men-born-blind.

'Aveugles' is very different. In it, *, whom many readers would have known to be the ex-convict author of the anonymous *Letter* referred to in the previous article, says nothing of the *Letter* or its blind men and instead gives a description of an Academy for the Blind in Japan, whose members win awards for their amazing feats of memory and their entertaining histories, recounted in verse and song.[22] Such an Academy did apparently exist – * refers to the Jesuit Père Charlevoix's *Histoire du Japon* [History of Japan] (1715) – but it is not impossible that it is also an ironic image of the group of Encyclopedists themselves whose history of knowledge would not be recorded orally but in many volumes of printed text. The editors are playing a game with each other and with any reader in the know.

What is most interesting about 'Aveugle' for our purposes here is that 0 says that the anonymous author of the *Letter* mentions a man-born-blind 'qu'il a connu, et qui vraisemblablement vit encore. Cet *aveugle* qui demeure au Puiseaux en Gâtinais, est chimiste et musicien.' [whom he knew and who is presumably still alive. This *blind man* who lives in Puiseaux in the Gâtinais, is a chemist and a musician.][23] Of course, this could be part of the game also – the adverb 'vraisemblablement' [presumably] is ambiguous, and the extra detail about the man-born-blind of Puiseaux being a musician is also taken from the *Letter*.[24] However, seemingly incontrovertible evidence that he was a real person and that the anonymous author of the *Letter*, whom we know to be Diderot and whom we also know to be *, knew him is to be found, most unexpectedly, in an article in the second volume of the *Encyclopédie* (1752) devoted to bonnet-making – 'Bonneterie'.[25]

The information for the article was provided by one 'Sieur Pichard', whom d'Alembert describes in the 'Discours préliminaire' [Preliminary Discourse] as a 'Marchand Fabriquant Bonnetier' [Bonnet-Maker and Seller].[26] The archives reveal that he worked on the rue Mouffetard in

22 'Aveugles', in *Encyclopédie*, vol. 1, p. 873.
23 'Aveugle', in *Encyclopédie*, vol. 1, p. 870.
24 DPV, 4, p. 25; Hobson and Harvey, p. 36; *Letter*, p. 178.
25 The second volume is dated 1751, but it appeared in January 1752. The article, 'Bonneterie', is on pp. 325–8. It is related to the article 'Bas' [Stocking] – one of Diderot's best known contributions to the *Encyclopédie*, see vol. 2, p. 98, and DPV, 6, p. 202–5.
26 D'Alembert, 'Discours préliminaire', in *Encyclopédie*, vol. 1, p. xliv.

the Latin quarter,[27] not far from where Diderot lived.[28] The final two paragraphs of the article are not by Pichard, however; they are preceded by '*', are written in the first person and contain a cross-reference to the article, 'Aveugle'. The asterisked final paragraphs read:

> * Je finirai cet article par un fait qui pourra être de quelqu'utilité à d'autres marchands bonnetiers qu'au sieur Pichard. Il est constant qu'il n'y a point de fouloire bien entretenue, qui ne consomme au moins pour dix sous d'eau par jour, et un marchand bonnetier peut avoir chez lui jusqu'à six, huit, dix fouloires, ce qui fait pour l'eau seulement un objet assez considérable. Le Sr Pichard parlait un jour de cette dépense, devant un aveugle de naissance déjà connu (dont il s'agit dans la *Lettre sur les aveugles* et dans l'art. Aveugle), et cet aveugle lui donna un conseil dont on ne s'était pas encore avisé depuis qu'on fait de la *bonneterie:* ce fut de se servir de l'eau de son puits; cela n'était pas difficile à trouver, diront ceux qui ignorent que l'eau de puits est très dure et se charge si difficilement de savon, qu'il n'est pas possible d'en faire usage en *bonneterie*. Mais notre aveugle savait très bien, par l'usage qu'il avait de la distillation, que cette même eau de puits distillée devenait très pénétrante, se chargeait de savon avec une extrême facilité, et en demandait même beaucoup moins que l'eau de rivière, pour produire le même effet.
>
> Il savait encore que le travail de la *bonneterie* demandait que l'on tint perpétuellement du feu sous la chaudière qui fournit de l'eau aux fouloires. Il conseilla donc au sieur Pichard de placer un grand alambic entre deux chaudières, qui recevraient l'eau qui s'en

---

27 According to the Minutes des Notaires de Paris (Archives Nationales), the Pichard family had been 'bonnetiers' on the rue Mouffetard since at least the early seventeenth century (according to the marriage certificate for Jean Pichart, 'bonnetier', ET/XVIII/250, dated 3 May 1637). The Pichard mentioned in 'Bonneterie' is likely to be either Charles or Jean Pichard, both 'marchands bonnetiers', living on the rue Mouffetard, though in different parishes, the former in the parish of Saint Étienne du Mont and the latter in that of Saint Médard. Notary documents show that on 19 January 1751, Charles became a 'maître et gardien en charge' in the Corporation des Bonnetiers [Guild of Bonnet-Makers] (ET/LXXXV/527), and that by April 1751, Jean had evidently died; a settlement of 28 April 1751 shows the ownership of the house on the rue Mouffetard being split equally between his son Jean-François, who continued to live there and continued the family business, and three daughters – Marie-Geneviève and Catherine, both married to 'marchands bonnetiers', and the unmarried Jeanne-Marguerite (ET/XVII/797).

28 In 1746, Diderot was living on the rue Mouffetard itself, see Diderot, *Correspondance*, Georges Roth (ed.), 16 volumes (Paris, Minuit, 1955–70), vol. 1, p. 53. By the end of 1748, he was living close by, just a little further west, on the rue de la Vieille-Estrapade (see Laurent Versini, 'Diderot, piéton à Paris'. *Travaux de Littérature*, 13 (2000), 117–94, p. 181).

distillerait, et qui la rendraient dans les fouloires. L'alambic de la fouloire du Sr Pichard est d'une forme singulière; il est concave en-dessous, et oppose une large surface au feu; il s'en élève perpétuellement une masse considérable de vapeurs; il est placé de façon qu'il est échauffé par le feu même qui entretient la chaleur des chaudières, et il fournit aux fouloires de l'eau qui ne coûte rien, qui épargne le savon, et qui foule mieux que l'eau de rivière.[29]

* I shall finish this article with a fact that could be useful to other bonnet-sellers besides Sieur Pichard. It is a simple fact that there is no working felting mill that does not use at least ten sous-worth of water a day, and a merchant can have as many as six, eight or ten mills, which makes the water alone a quite considerable expense. One day Mr Pichard was speaking of this expense in front of a man-born-blind who is known to us already (and is in the *Letter on the Blind* and the art. Blind Man), and this blind man gave him some advice that no one had thought of since bonnet-making began: he should use the water from his well. There's nothing remarkable about that, those people will say, who are unaware that well water is very hard and that it is so difficult to dissolve soap in it that it cannot be used in bonnet-making. But our blind man was well-versed in distillation and he knew full well that once distilled, the well-water would turn soft, lather very easily and require much less soap than the river water to obtain the same effect.

He also knew that bonnet-making required a constant flame beneath the furnace that heats the water for the felting mills. So he advised Mr Pichard to install a large still between two furnaces; the evaporated water would come into the still and be sent on to the mills. The still that Mr Pichard installed at his felting mill is a strange shape. It is concave underneath so that the greatest surface area is exposed to the flame. It constantly gives off lots of steam. It is positioned so as to be heated by the same flame that maintains the temperature of the furnaces, and it provides the mills with water which costs nothing, saves on soap and feels better than river water.

Now these details really are, as *** puts it in the *Letter*, 'not very philosophical'. Moreover, *'s narrative would seem to provide evidence that ***'s man-born-blind of Puiseaux knew 'some chemistry', did indeed sometimes come to Paris, and, most importantly, was 'not imaginary'. Here we see him applying his knowledge of chemistry and distillation to bonnet-making, a perfect example of the utilitarian value of knowledge

29 'Bonneterie', in *Encyclopédie*, vol. 2, p. 328.

that the *Encyclopédie* seeks to promote. So perhaps we should take at face value ***'s claim that the 'not very philosophical' details are there to make the reader decide that the man-born-blind of Puiseaux is 'not imaginary' – or perhaps we should take it as a double bluff.

The relative dates of composition of 'Bonnet-making' and the *Letter* are unknown: the article appeared after the *Letter* but it could have been written earlier. This uncertainty allows what is very probably just a simple – and amusing – coincidence to open up a tiny chink of doubt as to whether the man-born-blind of Puiseaux was in fact 'of Puiseaux': the phonetic echo between 'Puiseaux' and the advice we are told the man-born-blind gave to Pichard, namely that he should source his water from his own well, which is, in French, 'puiser de l'eau'.[30]

But why does *** raise the possibility that the man-born-blind of Puiseaux was imaginary in the first place? If *** had not said he was not imaginary, the reader might never have thought he was. The aim seems to be to encourage the reader to reflect on the judgements she makes of textual evidence and to make her just as aware of how easily she rejects what she is told as false as she is of how easily she might accept it to be true. Refusal to believe is as much a target here as gullibility, as it is all the way through the *Letter*.

Saunderson

Games of a related sort, if they are indeed games, are played in relation to the second man-born-blind to appear in the *Letter* – Saunderson. *** presents him in such a way that he resembles the man-born-blind of Puiseaux. Of the latter, we recall that 'his father taught philosophy to much acclaim in the University of Paris' and 'his love of pleasure [. . .] led him astray in his youth', and the same details appear in the reverse order with respect to Saunderson, of whom *** tells us, 'fut entraîné par son goût à l'étude des mathématiques' [his taste led him to study mathematics],[31] and 'professa les mathématiques dans l'université de Cambridge avec un succès étonnant' [was astonishingly successful at teaching mathematics in the University of Cambridge].[32] The two blind men are clearly set up to echo one other – one led by pleasure, the other by a love of maths; one with an academic father in philosophy at Paris, the other himself

30 Diderot sometimes draws attention to the possibility of names being comic. For example, the mention of a man named 'Odiot' in *Histoire de la peinture en cire* [History of Encaustic Painting] (1755) prompts the following footnote: 'Voilà un endroit sur lequel la plupart des lecteurs seront tentés de porter un faux jugement: je les en préviens.' [This is where the majority of readers will be tempted into making a wrong judgement; I warn them against doing so.] (DPV, IX, p. 158).

31 DPV, 4, p. 41; Hobson and Harvey, p. 53; *Letter*, p. 192.

32 DPV, 4, p. 42; Hobson and Harvey, p. 54; *Letter*, p. 194.

an academic in maths at Cambridge. And like the man-born-blind of Puiseaux, Saunderson combines fact and fiction.

There was a real Nicholas Saunderson: he held the prestigious Lucasian Chair of Mathematics at the University of Cambidge from 1711 until his death in 1739, a chair that had earlier been held by Newton (from 1669 until 1702). Saunderson had contracted smallpox as an infant, as a result of which he not only went blind but also lost his eyes, and his academic career was an unusual one. Having received some formal education, he arrived in Cambridge in 1707. He was not, however, a member of the University – he was simply staying in the rooms of one Joshua Dunn, a Fellow-Commoner of Christ's College, and during his stay, he set himself up as a 'Master', giving lessons in maths and particularly Newtonian science. When in 1711 Whiston was forced to resign from the Lucasian Chair for having expressed his heterodox religious views too openly, it was suggested that Saunderson, now a famous Master in Cambridge, be appointed to the Chair. He took up the post that year, but not before a special case had been made for him to be awarded a degree, a qualification he still did not hold but which – not unreasonably – the University statutes required of its Lucasian Chair.[33] These facts are known to us through a biographical essay entitled 'Memoirs of the Life and Character of Dr Nicholas Saunderson', prefixed to Saunderson's two-volume posthumously published *Elements of Algebra* (1740)[34] and written by his son, John, on the basis of details supplied by various friends of the deceased, many of them colleagues, fellows of various Cambridge Colleges. But how and what did Diderot know of Saunderson?

It is a question that has been asked by editors of the *Letter*,[35] though, in fact, it would have been far stranger had Diderot not known about him, for Saunderson was well known in France in philosophical and, in particular, Encyclopedist circles. Hobson and Harvey note that Voltaire mentioned the blind mathematician 'Saounderson', a common French spelling of his name, in his correspondence in the 1730s.[36] They could add that Voltaire even went as far as to adopt 'Sanderson le jeune' as a

---

33 The post is held today by Stephen Hawking. For a history of the Lucasian Chair, see Kevin C. Knox, *From Newton to Hawking: a History of Cambridge University's Lucasian Professors of Mathematics* (Cambridge: Cambridge University Press, 2003).

34 Nicholas Saunderson, *The Elements of Algebra, in Ten Books: by Nicholas Saunderson LL.D. Late Lucasian Professor of the Mathematics in the University of Cambridge, and Fellow of the Royal Society. To which is prefixed, an account of the author's life and character, collected from his oldest and most intimate acquaintances*, 2 volumes (Cambridge: Printed at the University-Press and sold by Mrs. Saunderson at Cambridge, by John Whiston bookseller at Boyle's Head in Fleet Street London, and Thomas Hammond in York, 1740).

35 Hobson and Harvey, p. 215.

36 Hobson and Harvey, pp. 215–6.

pseudonym at one stage in his correspondence concerning the publication and distribution of the *Lettres philosophiques* [Philosophical Letters] (1734), which involved various degrees of deceit and subterfuge. The name was perhaps chosen to suggest to his correspondent that he wished him to turn a blind eye to some aspects of his dealings.[37]

Hobson and Harvey also note that Voltaire's name appears in the list of subscribers to Saunderson's *Elements*.[38] They could add that it also lists one 'Mons. De Button', which is presumably an Anglophone typesetter's misprint for Buffon, who had a strong interest in Newtonian mathematics and had translated Newton's *Method of Fluxions*.[39] Not a great deal is known about Diderot's relations with Buffon before the *Letter*, though we know that in mid 1749 Diderot was reading the first volume of Buffon's *Histoire naturelle*. The third volume, which appeared later that year, contains a footnote praising the *Letter on the Blind*.[40]

The Encyclopedists also knew and thought highly of Saunderson's work: d'Alembert refers to the *Elements* in a number of articles and praises it as an excellent textbook.[41] Another mathematical contributor, La Chapelle, refers to Saunderson in his own textbook, *Institutions de géométrie* [Institutes of Geometry] (1746), in which he also explains that

---

37 Letter to Cideville, 10 June 1733. For more details of these dealings, see Nicholas Cronk, 'Voltaire and the Benefits of Censorship: The Example of the *Lettres philosophiques*', in E. Joe Johnson and Byron R. Wells (eds), *An American Voltaire: Essays in Memory of J. Patrick Lee* (Newcastle Upon Tyne: Cambridge Scholars Publishing, 2009), pp. 33–61.

38 Hobson and Harvey, p. 218.

39 Isaac Newton, *Méthode des fluxions et des suites infinies* (Paris: chez de Bure l'aîné, 1740).

40 It reads: 'On trouvera un grand nombre de faits très intéressants au sujet des aveugles-nés, dans un petit ouvrage qui vient de paraître, et qui a pour titre: *Lettre sur les aveugles, à l'usage de ceux qui voient*. L'auteur y a répandu partout une métaphysique très fine et très vraie, par laquelle il rend raison de toutes les différences que doit produire dans l'esprit d'un homme la privation absolue du sens de la vue.' [A large number of very interesting facts about men-born-blind can be found in a little work that has just appeared with the title, *Letter on the Blind for the use of those who can see*. The author has sprinkled throughout it a very subtle and very true philosophy that allows him to explain all the differences that the complete deprivation of the sense of sight must produce in the mind.] (Buffon, *Histoire naturelle*, vol. 3 (1749), p. 318). We should note that an almost identical phrase, 'la métaphysique est partout très fine et très vraie' [the philosophy is very subtle and very true throughout], is also to be found in the *Encyclopédie* article, 'Aveugle' (p. 870), which suggests that Buffon may have had access to the article before it was published; indeed we might wonder whether Buffon had actually read the *Letter* in 1749.

41 See articles, 'Algèbre' [Algebra], 'Arithmétique universelle' [Universal Arithmetic], 'Diophante' [Diophantus], 'Racine d'une équation' [Root of an Equation].

he came to know of Saunderson through the abbé Sallier,[42] the librarian at the Bibliothèque du Roi [King's Library], whom Diderot also knew.[43]

Yet Diderot had not simply heard of Saunderson, whether through Voltaire, Buffon, Sallier or the Encyclopedists, he had also read the 'Memoirs of the Life and Character of Dr. Nicholas Saunderson' rather carefully. The *Letter* makes frequent use of the 'Memoirs'; it reports that Saunderson was married to the daughter of a Mr Dickons, the rector of Boxworth in Cambridgeshire, had a son and daughter who were both still living, and that he could distinguish real from counterfeit medals by his touch.[44] It also explores, as we'll see, certain details from the 'Memoirs' such as his use of language, his 'peculiar felicity of expression in conveying his ideas to others',[45] and may base its claim that the blind have a more abstract way of thinking on the claim in the 'Memoirs' that 'the blind are by necessity more abstracted than others.'[46] These details appear in the *Letter* with no reference being made to the 'Memoirs', though that is certainly their source.

There are, however, other details that appear in the *Letter*, of which it is explicitly claimed that they do come from the 'Memoirs' when that is not the case. Such details primarily concern Saunderson's religious views. Whereas those that *** provided of the man-born-blind-of-Puiseaux's life were deliberately 'not very philosophical', those provided by almost everyone who knew Saunderson are not philosophical enough: 'Je suis bien fâché, Madame, que pour votre satisfaction et la mienne, on ne nous ait pas transmis de cet illustre aveugle plus de particularités intéressantes.

42 Jean-Baptiste de La Chapelle, *Institutions de géométrie*, third edition, 2 volumes (Paris: chez Debure l'Aîné, 1757), vol. 2, pp. 355–6. We do not know much about La Chapelle; Luneau de Boisjermain reports that Diderot did not think him a very reliable member of the *Encyclopédie* team (Frank A. Kafker, 'The Recruitment of the Encyclopedists'. *Eighteenth-Century Studies*, 6.4 (Summer, 1973), 452–61, p. 458). D'Alembert says La Chapelle told him he lost his faith after having read a number of clandestine works, such as the *Testament de Jean Meslier* (Jean Meslier, *Œuvres complètes*, Jean Deprun, Roland Desné, Albert Soboul (eds), 3 volumes (Paris: Editions Anthropos, 1970–72), vol 1. p. lxii); and most intriguingly, the police file on him records that he later said (on 20 June 1750) that it was he who gave Diderot the idea for Saunderson's deathbed speech, see Robert Darnton, 'Les Encyclopédistes et la police'. *Recherches sur Diderot et l'Encyclopédie*, 1 (1986), 94–109, p. 102.

43 Diderot had been regularly borrowing books from the library since 1747. See Jacques Proust, 'L'Initiation artistique de Diderot'. *Gazette des Beaux-Arts*, 55 (1960), 225–32. Anthony Strugnell lists four additional titles to those given by Proust, see 'Diderot chercheur: du nouveau sur les emprunts faits par Diderot à la Bibliothèque royale entre 1775 et 1782'. *Recherches sur Diderot et l'Encyclopédie*, 8 (1990), 12–19, p. 14, note 4.

44 Saunderson, 'Memoirs', in *Elements*, vol. 1, p. xii.

45 Saunderson, 'Memoirs', in *Elements*, vol. 1, p. iv.

46 Saunderson, 'Memoirs', in *Elements*, vol. 1, p. x.

[. . .] Il fallait que ceux qui vivaient avec lui fussent bien peu philosophes!' [I am rather upset to discover, Madame, that other interesting details from the life of this illustrious blind man have not been passed down to us for your satisfaction as well as mine. [. . .] How very unphilosophical those who lived with him must have been!].[47] Fortunately, however, there was someone, *** tells us – a 'disciple' of Saunderson, one William Inchlif – who was present at his master's bedside when he died and who recorded his final exchange with his vicar in a work entitled *The Life and Character of Dr. Nicholas Saunderson late Lucasian Professor of the Mathematicks in the University of Cambridge*, published in Dublin in 1747.[48] Outside the *Letter*, no trace of this work has been found. There was a bookseller and printer by the name of William Hinchliffe or Hinchcliffe,[49] but he was based in London, not Dublin, and there is no evidence that he wrote or printed a work with that title. Though it is hard to be certain of anything with respect to the *Letter*, it would appear that Inchlif's *Life and Character* is a hoax.

As hoaxes go, however, it is not an unphilosophical one. We'll explore it later. Here it is important simply to note that the relationship between the account of Saunderson's death in the 'Memoirs' and that found in the *Letter* is not best understood as a simple one between fact and fiction. Instead, his fictional final words are a kind of 'supplement' to the facts, purporting simply to supply text that was omitted from the original, but in so doing exaggerating ambiguities in the original and even calling its claims into question.[50] As we'll see, the effect of reading Inchlif's *Life and Character* is to make the 'Memoirs' appear retrospectively incomplete and dependent on the *Life and Character*, the contents of which not only supplement the 'Memoirs' but also reveal its inconsistencies. That is not to say that the *Life and Character* does not contain ambiguities of its own, and faced with these, the reader must apply her judgement and supply the meaning.

So both Saunderson and the man-born-blind of Puiseaux are located in a zone between fact and fiction, a zone we might think of, in Saunderson's case, as supplementary. Things are perhaps no less complicated in the case of the man-born-blind of Puiseaux, however, since when *** raises

---

47 DPV, 4, p. 53; Hobson and Harvey, p. 64; *Letter*, p. 203.

48 For a reading of Inchlif as a figure of the philosopher, see Pierre Hartmann, *Diderot. La figuration du philosophe* (Paris: José Corti, 2003), pp. 64–5.

49 Hobson and Harvey, p. 182, note 68.

50 It is a technique that Diderot would often use (see, for example, his *Supplément au Voyage de Bougainville* [Supplement to Bougainville's *Voyage*] (1772)). For the idea of the supplement in the work of Rousseau, see Jacques Derrida, *De la grammatologie* (Paris: Minuit, 1967) and *Of Grammatology*, Gayatri Spivak (trans.) (Baltimore: Johns Hopkins University Press, 1976).

the possibility, even as he denies it, that the blind man is imaginary, in addition to asking her to consider her own gullibility and/or incredulity, he points to the possibility that Madame might recognize the blind man from elsewhere – not from the bonnet-maker's on the rue Mouffetard, but from literary and philosophical texts she might have read. It is to these men-born-blind that we now turn, noting that if we think of the man-born-blind of Puiseaux as standing in a long line of men-born-blind, another play on the word 'Puiseaux' might be heard: when the blind lead the blind in the French version of the Biblical proverb, they fall into a 'puits'.

Two

The Blind Leading the Blind Leading the Blind Leading the Blind Leading the Blind . . .

We noted earlier Farrell's erroneous claim that the man-born-blind of Puiseaux was called 'Lenôtre' and observed that it might nonetheless be instructive because it highlights the *Letter*'s frequent use of the first-person plural possessive pronoun in relation to the man-born-blind of Puiseaux. That frequency is not without significance when we consider that pronouns are relational: 'ours' gains meaning in relation to 'theirs'; 'our blind man' depends on 'theirs'.[1] So who might 'they' and 'their man-born-blind' be?

Molyneux's Man-Born-Blind

At one level, *** is seeking to distinguish the man-born-blind of Puiseaux from Réaumur's girl-born-blind. However, critics have been wrong to think that ***'s lack of interest in Réaumur's spectacle (and Réaumur's alleged interest in *** not being there to witness it) signals that Molyneux's Problem is pushed to one side until the final section of the *Letter*, where it is explicitly discussed in detail.[2] Certainly it is true that *** does digress, and indeed he calls the reader's attention to his digressions more than once,[3] but the *Letter*'s treatment of Molyneux's Problem is not confined to the beginning and end. What makes it hard to recognize as such is the fact that it simply does not resemble that of his predecessors and contemporaries (nor indeed that of his successors).

Molyneux's Problem opens, we recall, by instructing the reader to

---

1 For Diderot's later use of pronouns, see Marian Hobson, 'Deictics and Dialectics in the *Neveu de Rameau*', in Hobson, *Diderot and Rousseau*, pp. 115–25.

2 See, for example, Marie-Hélène Chabut, 'La *Lettre sur les aveugles*: l'écriture comme écart'. *SVEC*, 304 (1992), 1245–9; Daniel Brewer, *The Discourse of Enlightenment in Eighteenth-Century France: Diderot and the Art of Philosophizing* (Cambridge: Cambridge University Press, 1993), pp. 98–107.

3 DPV, 4, pp. 45, 66; Hobson and Harvey, pp. 57, 77; *Letter*, pp. 197, 214.

'suppose a Man born blind and now adult and taught by his touch.' It is only once we have already supposed him to be in possession of ideas gained through haptic experience that Molyneux instructs us to suppose him 'made to see'. All Diderot's predecessors, contemporaries and successors – Locke, Leibniz, Berkeley, Voltaire, La Mettrie, Maupertuis, Condillac, Turgot, Mérian, Reid – gloss over the first supposition and fast-forward to the second, beginning their treatment of the Problem at the moment when the man-born-blind is made to see. By contrast, Diderot devotes serious attention to the first supposition by having *** go to Puiseaux and see what the sense of touch would have taught a man-born-blind 'and now adult' about the world. Réaumur's alleged refusal does not only permit *** to converse rather than spectate, it also enables him to work through Molyneux's Problem stage by stage, starting right at the very beginning before the man is made to see.

Some confirmation that the man-born-blind of Puiseaux may be thought of as ***'s response to Molyneux's initial injunction to suppose can be found at the end of the story of the visit to Puiseaux, where we read, 'Première question. Comment un aveugle-né se forme-t-il des idées des figures?' [Question one. How does a man-born-blind form ideas of shapes?].[4] This question seems to have perplexed the editors of the *Letter* in Diderot's *Œuvres complètes* [Complete Works] as they insert a footnote stating that the text is inconsistent because 'Question one' is not followed by a 'Question two'.[5] Yet 'Question two' must be Molyneux's question to the ex-blind man, found in the second stage of the Problem. The *Letter*'s two-stage treatment is disconcerting because it does what no other philosophers do, namely establish what ideas a man-born-blind can gain from touch. It is this that is established, as we'll see, in conversation with the man-born-blind of Puiseaux.

Such a treatment of the Problem might seem perverse in that it devotes so much time to the initial supposition, one that other philosophers took to be a mere preliminary. It might be thought of as comic, even proto-Sternean: just as it will take the eponymous narrator of Sterne's novel, *Tristram Shandy* (1759), three volumes to arrive at the moment when he is born, so it takes *** two-thirds of his letter to arrive at the moment when a man-born-blind gets to see. And yet the attention given to what other philosophers have thought of as mere 'back story' will turn out to have some important philosophical implications and perhaps some moral ones too.

Molyneux's is not the only man-born-blind with whom the *Letter* has a relationship. I explore here the men-born-blind who appear in works by Sextus Empiricus, Montaigne, Descartes, Gassendi and La Mothe

---

4 DPV, 4, p. 29; Hobson and Harvey, p. 39; *Letter*, p. 181.
5 DPV, 4, p. 29, note 32.

Le Vayer, but my exploration begins with the blind man who first appeared as a comic type in medieval farce. He has not been given a role in the *Letter* before but he deserves attention, for although there are numerous differences between him and the blind men of the *Letter*, there are also significant echoes.

A Comic Type

This blind man – perhaps he was born blind, perhaps he went blind – is to be found in a number of medieval and early modern texts that represent the blind as marginal figures, outcasts, itinerants and beggars.[6] As such, the blind man has a dual status and is associated both with the pauper or pilgrim, eliciting pity, sympathy and alms, and with the drunkard, the lecher and the thief, and many texts play on that duality for comic and satirical effect.

In the anonymous Spanish picaresque novel, *Lazarillo de Tormes* (1554, French translation 1560),[7] for example, a boy named Lazaro (his name of course evoking another group with whom the blind are often associated – the lame) goes into the service of a blind man as his guide. His master's blindness figures his defective morality: he is a lying, cheating, cruel and miserly religious hypocrite. When his young guide misleads and outwits him, the reader can only approve. The novel is probably partly based on an anonymous, thirteenth-century French farce, *Le Garçon et l'aveugle* [The Boy and the Blind Man], in which the blind man was also a rogue and a hypocrite, feigning piety to receive alms, of which he in fact has no need since he is a rich miser.[8] And it is not just piety and poverty that he feigns, but also his blindness. This is a classic topos of farce to this day, and it was present on the early modern French stage in, for example, Le Grand's *L'Aveugle clairvoyant* [The Clear-Sighted Blind Man] (1716), in which the hero's blindness permits the 'wrong' hands to be held and 'wrong' faces to be slapped, and ludicrously unconvincing voices to be put on.[9]

The blind men in the *Letter* are genuinely blind, but the figure of the comic blind man is not as absent from the text as critical studies have tended either implicitly or explicitly to suggest. Certainly, Diderot's blind

6 See Weygand, *The Blind in French Society*, pp. 11–23; Kahren Jones Hellerstedt, 'The Blind Man and his Guide'. *Netherlands Quarterly for the History of Art*, 13.3/4 (1983), 163–81.

7 *Lazarillo de Tormes*, in *Lazarillo de Tormes and The Swindler: Two Spanish Picaresque Novels*, Michael Alpert (trans. intro. and notes) (London: Penguin, 2003), p. 10.

8 *Le garçon et l'aveugle: jeu du XIIIe siècle*, Jean Dufournet (trans. ed. and comm.) (Paris: Champion, 2007).

9 Marc-Antoine Le Grand, *L'aveugle clairvoyant* in M. Claude-Bernard Petitot, *Répertoire du théâtre français*, 23 volumes (Paris: Didot l'aîné, 1803–4), vol. 18, pp. 356–406. It is based on an earlier play (1650) of the same name by Brosse. I am grateful to Christian Biet for this reference.

men are not social outcasts – far from it – nor are they thieving, miserly, drunken religious hypocrites. However, they do hold moral and religious views that might be thought highly dubious and, moreover, the man-born-blind of Puiseaux (whose very absence of name may suggest a link to the comic type) is, as we'll see, as inclined to theft and an apparently innocent grope as his comic counterparts. Furthermore, there are many occasions on which *** himself might be said to feign blindness.

Yet Diderot's blind men are also hybrids. They combine aspects of farce with features of the sceptical commonplace, to which we now turn.

Sextus Empiricus's Man Who Sees and Hears Nothing

If Molyneux's 'man-born-blind and . . . made to see' has been said to be the emblem of the Enlightenment, the emblem of scepticism might be said to be a man-born-blind who, in not seeing, shows us that we too might be blind. He is to be found in the first instance, and in a slightly more disabled state, being deaf as well as blind, in Sextus Empiricus's *Outlines of Scepticism*.

Sextus Empiricus presents the reader with ten 'modes' or ways of arguing that are designed to induce the reader to suspend her judgement. His man-born-blind-and-deaf appears in the third thought-experiment, which goes as follows:

> Let us conceive of someone who from birth has touch, smell and taste, but who sees and hears nothing. He will suppose that there is nothing visible or audible, and that there exist only those kinds of quality that he is able to grasp. So it is possible that we too, having only the five senses, grasp from among the qualities of the apple only those we are capable of grasping, although other qualities can exist, impressing other sense-organs, in which we have no share, so that we do not grasp the objects perceptible by them.[10]

Sextus is asking the reader to imagine a blind and deaf man who is unable to imagine either seeing or hearing, who cannot imagine that the apple he can feel, taste and smell is red or green and makes a crunching noise when he bites into it. And he asks us to see a version of ourselves in this blind and deaf man: just as he is unaware of his limitations, so we might be unaware of ours. It is after all possible that the apple has qualities we cannot grasp and which we are as unable to imagine as the blind and deaf man cannot imagine colour and sound. And since we cannot be certain that the knowledge we gain from our senses is more than merely partial,

---

10 Sextus Empiricus, *Outlines of Scepticism*, Julia Annas and Jonathan Barnes (ed. and trans.) (Cambridge: Cambridge University Press, 2000), pp. 26–7.

we must, Sextus tells us, suspend our judgement. As Derrida has put it in the opening lines of his *Mémoires d'aveugle* [Memoirs of the Blind] (1994):

> Avant que le doute ne devienne un système, la *skepsis* est chose des yeux, le mot désigne une perception visuelle, l'observation, la vigilance, l'attention du regard au cours de l'examen. On guette, on réfléchit à ce qu'on voit, on réfléchit ce qu'on voit en retardant le moment de conclure.[11]

> Before doubt becomes a system, *skepsis* is about the eyes. The word refers to a visual perception, to observation, vigilance, careful visual scrutiny. You're on the look-out, you reflect on what you see, you reflect what you see by postponing the moment when you draw a conclusion.[12]

Sextus Empiricus's man-born-blind-and-deaf, along with the self-reflexive gaze that imagining oneself observing him engenders, appears in a number of early modern French texts such as Charron's *De la Sagesse* [Of Wisdom] (1601) and Cyrano de Bergerac's *Voyage dans la lune* [Journey to the Moon] (1657). Charron says:

> Nous vivons très commodément avec cinq, et peust-estre qu'il nous en manque encore un, ou deux, ou trois; mais ne se peust sçavoir: un sens ne peust descouvrir l'autre; et s'il en manque un par nature, l'on ne le sçauroit trouver à dire. L'homme né aveugle, ne sçauroit jamais concevoir qu'il ne void pas, ny desirer de voir ou regretter la veuë, il dira bien peust estre, qu'il voudra voir: mais cela vient qu'il a ouy dire ou apprins d'autruy, qu'il a à dire quelque chose. La raison est que les sens sont les premieres portes et entrées à la cognoissance. Ainsi l'homme ne pouvant imaginer plus que les cinq qu'il a, il ne sçauroit deviner s'il y en a davantage en nature, mais il y en peut avoir.[13]

---

11 Jacques Derrida, *Mémoires d'aveugle: l'autoportrait et autres ruines* (Paris: Réunion des Musées Nationaux, 1991), p. 9.

12 Jacques Derrida, *Memoirs of the Blind: The Self-Portrait and other Ruins*, Pascale-Anne Brault and Michael Naas (trans.) (Chicago: University of Chicago Press, 1993), p. 1 (translation modified). Derrida's interest is in faith, which he sees as suspending or, rather, definitively bringing to an end the sceptical suspension of judgement.

13 Pierre Charron, *Toutes les Œuvres de Pierre Charron, Parisien, Docteur es Droicts, Chantre et Chanoine Theologal de Condom. Dernière edition. Reveuës, corrigées & augmentées*, 2 volumes (Paris: Jacques Villery, 1635), vol. 1, p. 35. Charron's text echoes Montaigne, as we'll see.

> We live very comfortably with five senses, and perhaps we are missing one or two or three; but we are unable to know whether this is the case because one sense cannot discover the other, and if we are naturally missing one, we could not find it out to say so. The man-born-blind could never conceive of what he lacks or desire to see or regret his lack of sight. He might perhaps say he would like to see, but that comes only from having heard or learnt from others that he is to say something. This is because the senses are the primary gateways and entrances for knowledge. Since man is therefore unable to imagine more than the five senses he has, he cannot imagine there to be more in nature, but there might be.

And an inhabitant of the moon informs Cyrano's astronaut that he, unlike his earthly counterpart, can feel the pull of the moon on the tides, sense iron as a magnet can, and knows what happens to animals once they have died. His earthly visitor is, by contrast, comparable to:

> un aveugle-né [qui] ne saurait s'imaginer ce que c'est que la beauté d'un paysage, le coloris d'un tableau, les nuances de l'iris; ou bien il se les figurera tantôt comme quelque chose de palpable, tantôt comme un manger, tantôt comme un son, tantôt comme une odeur. Tout de meme, si je voulais vous expliquer ce que je perçois par les sens qui vous manquent, vous vous le représenteriez comme quelque chose qui peut être ouï, vu, touché, fleuré ou savouré, et ce n'est rien cependant de tout cela.[14]

> a man-born-blind [who] cannot imagine the beauty of the landscape, the colours of a painting, or the tints of the rainbow. Or else he will imagine them sometimes as something palpable, sometimes as something edible, sometimes as a sound, sometimes as an odour. Likewise, if I tried to explain to you what I perceive through the senses you lack, you would imagine them as something which can be heard, seen, touched smelled, or tasted – and yet it is nothing of the kind.[15]

It is noteworthy that in each of these two cases, Sextus's man has acquired the sense of hearing. This no doubt reflects the primacy of vision in much early modern culture, and the related view that blindness was a greater

---

14 Cyrano de Bergerac, *L'Autre monde: ou, Les états et empire de la lune* in *Œuvres complètes*, Madeleine Alcover (ed.), 3 volumes (Paris: Champion, 2000), vol. 1, p. 64; see also pp. 150–1.

15 Cyrano de Bergerac, *Journey to the Moon*, Andrew Brown (trans.) (London: Hesperus, 2007), p. 39 (translation slightly modified); see also p. 110.

handicap than deafness made it sufficient for the purposes of the sceptical argument. Moreover, the conception of cognition on a visual model meant that self-reflexivity was conceived as involving looking rather than listening to oneself.

These are not the only implications of the sceptical blind and deaf man's acquisition of hearing, however. In other texts, it enables him to engage in conversation and to listen to the sighted, and also to speak to them and tell them about what it is he can do despite and sometimes because of his disabled state. It enables his observers to hear his point of view. As a result, the man-born-blind starts to take on an independent life of his own, one that is irreducible to the teachings of scepticism. His most significant walking, talking avatar is to be found in Montaigne's 'Apologie de Raimond Sebond' [Apology for Raimond Sebond] in the *Essais* [Essays] (1580–95).[16]

Montaigne's Gentleman of a Good House, Born Blind

The *Essais* contain a number of references to blind men and women and even to guide dogs for the blind, as well as some discussion of Montaigne's own ailing sight.[17] The most important and sustained discussion of blindness is to be found in the 'Apologie', where the essayist affirms that all our knowledge comes from our senses but expresses some doubt that we are in possession of them all.[18] Echoing Sextus Empiricus in order to persuade the reader of this doubt, he introduces a man-born-blind:

> Il est impossible de faire concevoir à un homme naturellement aveugle qu'il n'y void pas, impossible de luy faire desirer la veue

---

16 Some discussion of the relevance of Montaigne's discussion to the *Letter* can be found in Jerome Schwartz, *Diderot and Montaigne*, pp. 31–4, and in Francine Markovits, 'Mérian, Diderot et l'aveugle', in J. -B. Mérian, *Sur le Problème de Molyneux*, with a postface by Francine Markovits (Paris: Flammarion, 1984), pp. 225–7. See also my 'The Judgement of Experience: Seeing and Reading in Diderot's *Lettre sur les aveugles*', *French Studies*, 62.4 (2008), 404–16, and 'Pré-histoire d'un emblème des Lumières: l'aveugle-né de Montaigne à Diderot', in *Les Lumières en mouvement: la circulation des idées au XVIIIe siècle*, Isabelle Moreau (ed.), (Lyon: ENS, 2009), pp. 173–97.

17 In 'De ne contrefaire le malade' [Not to counterfeit being sick], Montaigne tells the story, taken from Seneca, of a blind woman who is unaware she has gone blind (Michel de Montaigne, *Essais*, Villey-Saulner (ed.) (Paris: Presses Universitaires de France, 2004), p. 689; *Essays*, in *The Complete Works*, Donald M. Frame (trans.) Stuart Hampshire (intro.) (London: Everyman, 2003), p. 634). It might be compared with his account of his own refusal or inability to accept his own diminishing capacities in 'De l'Expérience' [Of Experience] (*Essais*, p. 1105; *Essays*, pp. 1,033–4). The reference to guide dogs for the blind is to be found in the 'Apologie' (*Essais*, p. 463; *Essays*, pp. 412–3).

18 *Essais*, p. 588; *Essays*, p. 540.

> et regretter son defaut. Parquoy nous ne devons prendre aucune asseurance de ce que nostre ame est contente et satisfaicte de ceux que nous avons, veu qu'elle n'a pas dequoy sentir en cela sa maladie et son imperfection, si elle y est.[19]

> It is impossible to make a man who was born blind conceive that he does not see; impossible to make him desire sight and regret its absence. Wherefore we should take no assurance from the fact that our soul is content and satisfied with those senses we have, seeing that it has no means of feelings its malady and imperfection therein, if any there be.[20]

As in the ancient Greek text, the blind man reveals to the reader that she may be defective too, but the manner in which Montaigne makes his point is significantly different. Whereas Sextus suggests that we conceive of someone who cannot see, Montaigne states that we cannot make a man-born-blind conceive that he cannot see. This is a significant shift in perspective: Sextus was conducting a thought-experiment amongst the sighted in which the blind man was a silent object, whereas Montaigne suggests the possibility of a dialogue between the reader and a real blind man. Although such a dialogue is a failure because the blind man is deaf to the sighted person's attempts to make him conceive his lack, the possibility of communication between blind and sighted is nonetheless opened up. This possibility becomes more significant as the text goes on, as Montaigne makes the move that inaugurates the tradition in which the *Letter on the Blind* will later be found: he introduces a particular man-born-blind, whom he has himself actually seen.

Montaigne writes:

> J'ay veu un gentil-homme de bonne maison, aveugle nay, au-moins aveugle de tel aage qu'il ne sçait que c'est que veue: il entend si peu ce qui luy manque, qu'il use et se sert comme nous des paroles propres au voir, et les applique d'une mode toute sienne et particuliere. On luy presentoit un enfant du quel il estoit parrain; l'ayant pris entre ses bras: Mon Dieu, dict-il, le bel enfant! qu'il le faict beau voir! qu'il a le visage guay! Il dira comme l'un d'entre nous: Cette sale a une belle veue: il faict clair, il faict beau soleil. Il y a plus: car, par ce que ce sont nos exercices que la chasse, la paume, la bute, et qu'il l'a ouy dire, il s'y affectionne et s'y embesoigne, et croid y avoir la mesme part que nous y avons; il s'y picque et s'y plaist, et ne les

19 *Essais*, p. 589.
20 *Essays*, p. 540.

> reçoit pourtant que par les oreilles. On luy crie que voylà un lièvre, quand on est en quelque belle splanade où il puisse picquer; et puis on luy dict encore que voylà un lièvre pris: le voylà aussi fier de sa prise, comme il oit dire aux autres qu'ils le sont. L'esteuf, il le prend à la main gauche et le pousse à tout sa raquette; de la harquebouse, il en tire à l'adventure, et se paye de ce que ses gens luy disent qu'il est ou haut ou costié. Que sçait-on si le genre humain faict une sottise pareille, à faute de quelque sens, et que par ce defaut la plus part du visage des choses nous soit caché?[21]

> I have seen a gentleman of a good house, born blind, or at least blind from such an age that he does not know what sight is. He understands so little what he lacks, that he uses and employs as we do words appropriate to sight, and applies them in a manner all private and his own. He was presented with a boy, whose godfather he was; taking him in his arms, he said: 'My, what a handsome boy! How good it is to see him! What a gay face he has!' He will say like one of us: 'This room has a fine view; it is a clear day, the sun is shining bright.' There is more; for because hunting, tennis, and shooting are our sports, and he has heard this, he is fond of them and keenly interested in them, and thinks he has the same share in them that we do; he finds excitement and pleasure in them, and yet he takes them in only through his ears. They call to him that there goes a hare when they are in a bit of fine open country where he can spur his horse; and then they tell him later that there is a hare caught; and he is as proud of his catch as he hears the others say they are. The tennis ball he takes in his left hand and strokes with his racket; with the harquebus he shoots at random, and gets his fun by having his men tell him that he is either over or beside the mark. What do we know about whether mankind is doing something equally foolish for lack of some sense, and whether by this lack the greater part of the face of things is hidden from us?[22]

Sextus's purely hypothetical and abstract thought experiment ('let us conceive') has become concrete fact ('I have seen'), and the ancient Greek blind and deaf man has acquired, along with his sense of hearing, a social status, a godson, a love of the sporting life and ideas above his station. He has no idea what 'handsome', 'gay', 'fine view' and 'shining bright' actually mean, but he appropriates them for himself. He thinks he can play a sport like tennis that requires hand–eye coordination, or go hunting,

---

21 *Essais*, p. 589.
22 *Essays*, p. 541.

which requires the sportsman to train his eye on a target. Just as we settle in to feeling superior, however, Montaigne makes us laugh on the other side of our faces by pointing out that the claims we make about the world may very well be just like the blind man's tennis balls: so many shots in the dark. As we'll see, the *Letter* is full of such reflexive moves in which we are invited to see ourselves in the mirror of the blind.

Yet if we compare Montaigne's anecdote to Sextus's exemplum, it seems rather excessive: for the purpose of making the reader suspend her judgement on knowledge gained from the senses, all these details about a good house, a hare, a horse and a tennis ball are totally unnecessary. They are surplus to philosophical demand. There is, as Richard Scholar has observed, 'no need for us to know that he picks up tennis balls in his *left* hand'.[23] So what are they doing there?

Diderot would no doubt have called them 'not very philosophical' and claimed that they were included to make the reader judge the man not to be imaginary. And indeed we can be sure that this 'gentleman of a good house, born blind' was not imaginary: he is referred to in a number of other texts of the period which permit us to identify him as Monsieur de Guiméné, très-grand Seigneur de Bretagne et d'Anjou.[24] Moreover, (right-handed) tennis players do indeed hold the ball in their left hand.[25] Yet Montaigne's excessive details have another purpose besides this. Certainly we are encouraged to some extent to see the 'gentleman of a good house, born blind' as slightly ridiculous, farcical, as he goes around randomly firing his harquebus, and the inversion of the usual master-servant relation is definitely comic, but the anecdote may also be read another way.

Montaigne gives us so much information about the blind man's life that for the length of the anecdote we move away from seeing him as a blind and silent sign to be deciphered by the sighted (as he was in Sextus) to seeing the world through his blind eyes. For all that he is 'born blind', this 'gentleman of a good house' is coping perfectly well. This is no doubt why he is first called a 'gentleman of a good house' and only secondarily is he said to be 'born blind'. The sense of hearing is sufficient.

---

23 See Richard Scholar, *The Je-Ne-Sais-Quoi in Early Modern Europe: Encounters with a Certain Something* (Oxford, Oxford University Press, 2005), p. 246.

24 See Ambroise Paré, *Les Œuvres d'Ambroise Paré, conseiller et premier chirurgien du roy, divisées en vingt-sept livres: avec les figures et portraicts tant de l'Anatomie que des instruments de chirurgie et de plusieurs monstres: reveuz et augmentez par l'autheur pour la seconde édition* (Paris: Gabriel Buon, 1579), p. 715; Pierre de Bourdeille, Seigneur de Brantôme, *Discours sur les colonels de l'infanterie de France*, Etienne Vaucheret (ed.) preface by V. -L. Saulnier (Paris: Vrin, 1973), p. 144; Jucquel Rougeart, *Œuvres complètes (1578)*, Catherine Magnien-Simonin (ed.) (Geneva: Droz, 1988), p. 100.

25 I am grateful to Wes Williams for this observation.

It is no doubt not for nothing either that hunting is his chosen sport, as it is one for which the sense of hearing is crucial.[26] Hearing is also crucial for speech and, although it is said that the manner in which he uses the words 'handsome', 'gay' and 'fine' is 'all private and his own', he is, in fact, using them in a way that is all public and shared by everyone. We all say babies are handsome and the view is fine; language functions perfectly well without visual referents underpinning it. Such phrases are the mark of polite society and, as such, a blind man who is educated and cultivated is as capable of uttering them correctly as the sighted. And so, the blind man who we thought was supposed to be demonstrating the idea that we should not trust the knowledge we gain from our senses because it might very well be partial suggests something rather different.

In Montaigne's expanded version of Sextus's thought-experiment, the man-born-blind is doing fine, shooting hares and saying all the right things at all the right moments. While it may be impossible to make him conceive of the advantages of sight, it is perfectly possible for him to make the sighted conceive of life without sight. As long as you have hearing (and a social station that enables you to have plenty of servants), it is totally unnecessary. Indeed, as the first of the epigraphs to this essay states, Montaigne would himself rather have forgone his own sense of sight than lost his hearing and with it, the pleasure of conversation.

Montaigne's man-born-blind was well known to many early modern readers. As we'll see, Diderot had certainly read the story, as a number of echoes in the *Letter* reveal. Moreover, he was not the only one in the 1740s to associate the gentleman of a good house with Saunderson: Le Blanc's *Lettres d'un Français* [Letters from a Frenchman] (1745) reports that the blind Professor of Mathematics at the University of Cambridge enjoys hunting:

> Mais qui croirait que la Chasse pût faire le plus grand plaisir d'un philosophe et d'un philosophe aveugle! Tel est cependant le cas du célèbre Sanderson [sic], Professeur de Mathématique à Cambridge: le malheur qu'il a d'avoir perdu la vûe, ne l'empêche ni de donner des leçons d'optique, ni de courir après un renard. Son cheval est accoutumé à suivre celui de son valet: ce n'est pas seulement l'exercice qu'il aime; le bruit des chiens et des chasseurs le transporte, il en fait lui-même autant que tout le reste de son équipage. Montaigne parle d'un aveugle-né, qui avait le même goût pour la chasse. *Voilà un lièvre pris,* dit-il; *le voilà aussi fier de sa prise, comme il oït dire aux autres qu'ils le sont.* Nous ne devons notre bonheur qu'à

26 See, for example, Jacques du Fouilloux, *La Vénerie* (Poitiers, 1561). I am grateful to Milad Doueihi for this reference.

> notre imagination: qu'il est heureux d'en avoir une qui se satisfait à si peu de frais.[27]

> But who would believe that hunting could be the greatest pleasure of a philosopher and a blind philosopher at that! Yet such is the case of the famous Sanderson [sic], Professor of Mathematics at Cambridge: the misfortune of having lost his sight prevents him neither from giving lectures on optics nor from chasing a fox. His horse is accustomed to following his valet's; but it's not only the exercise he likes: the sound of the dogs and the other hunters transports him, and he makes as much as the whole of the rest of the company. Montaigne speaks of a man-born-blind with the same taste for hunting. *There is a hare caught*, he says; *and he is as proud of his catch as he hears the others say they are*. We owe our happiness to our imagination alone; how fortunate he is to have one that is satisified at such little expense.

There is no hint of fox hunting in either Saunderson's 'Memoirs' or in the *Letter* but, as we'll see, the man-born-blind of Puiseaux is, amongst other things, an excellent shot. He is also a walking, talking version of an analogy that appears in Descartes' *La Dioptrique* [Dioptrics] (1637), and it is to that text that we now turn.

Descartes's Analogy

In order to explain the phenomena of both sight and light, Descartes makes particularly striking – and deliberately paradoxical – use of an analogy with a man-born-blind. It appears twice in *La Dioptrique*. In the first chapter, he asks the reader to recall those occasions on which he has been walking in the dark and needed a stick to guide him:

> Il vous est bien sans doute arrivé quelquefois, en marchant de nuit sans flambeau par des lieux un peu difficiles, qu'il fallait vous aider d'un bâton pour vous conduire, et vous avez pour lors pu remarquer que vous sentiez, par l'entremise de ce bâton, les divers objets qui se rencontraient autour de vous, et même que vous pouviez distinguer s'il y avait des arbres, ou des pierres, ou du sable, ou de l'eau, ou de l'herbe, ou de la boue, ou quelque autre chose de semblable. Il est vrai que cette sorte de sentiment est un peu confuse et obscure, en ceux qui n'en ont pas un long usage; mais considérez-la en ceux qui, étant nés aveugles, s'en sont servis toute leur vie, et vous l'y trouverez si parfaite et si exacte, qu'on pourrait quasi dire qu'ils

27 Jean-Bernard Le Blanc, *Lettres d'un Français*, 2 volumes (The Hague: Jean Neaulme, 1745), vol. 2, p. 153. The work is closely modelled on Voltaire's *Lettres philosophiques*.

voient des mains, ou que leur bâton est l'organe de quelque sixième sens, qui leur a été donné au défaut de la vue.[28]

No doubt you have had the experience of walking at night over rough ground without a light, and finding it necessary to use a stick in order to guide yourself. You may then have been able to notice that by means of this stick you could feel the various objects situated around you, and that you could even tell whether they were trees or stones or sand or water or grass or mud or any other such thing. It is true that this kind of sensation is somewhat confused and obscure in those who do not have long practice of it. But consider it in those born blind, who have made use of it all their lives: with them, you will find, it is so perfect and so exact that one might almost say that they see with their hands, or that their stick is the organ of some sixth sense given to them in place of sight.[29]

These two ideas, seeing with hands and sensing with a stick, form the basis for Descartes's understanding of visual perception, which is designed to counter any theory according to which visual perception is representational (haptic impressions do not look like their objects) and, in particular, the Epicurean claim that objects emit simulacra. Whether his theory is accepted or not, his paradoxical notion of 'seeing with hands' has an afterlife in a number of texts, including the *Letter*.[30]

For all his analogies between sight and touch, Descartes is not interested in haptic perception as such, however, and certainly does not hold that it provides more accurate knowledge than sight. Instead, once the analogy has served its purpose of undermining other theories of vision, he abandons sensible qualities in favour of a conception of vision as a form of geometrical reasoning. The blind man and his sticks do not disappear, however, since in a further striking comparison, Descartes represents the geometrical conception itself by an image of a blind man holding two sticks in such a way as their ends touch.

---

28 René Descartes, *Œuvres de Descartes*, Charles Adam and Paul Tannery (eds), 11 volumes (Paris: Vrin, 1964–76), vol. 6, pp. 83–4.

29 René Descartes, *The Philosophical Writings of Descartes*, John Cottingham, Robert Stoothoff and Dugald Murdoch (trans.), 3 volumes (Cambridge: Cambridge University Press, 1985), vol. 1, p. 153.

30 In Marana's *L'Espion turc* [The Turkish Spy], a blind man who can discern the colour of silk by touching it is said to be one of the wonders of Paris and of nature. See Giovanni Paolo Marana, *L'Espion turc dans les cours des princes chrétiens, ou lettres et mémoires d'un envoyé secret de la Porte dans les cours de l'Europe*, 7 volumes (Londres: Aux dépens de la Compagnie, 1742), vol. 2, pp. 285–6.

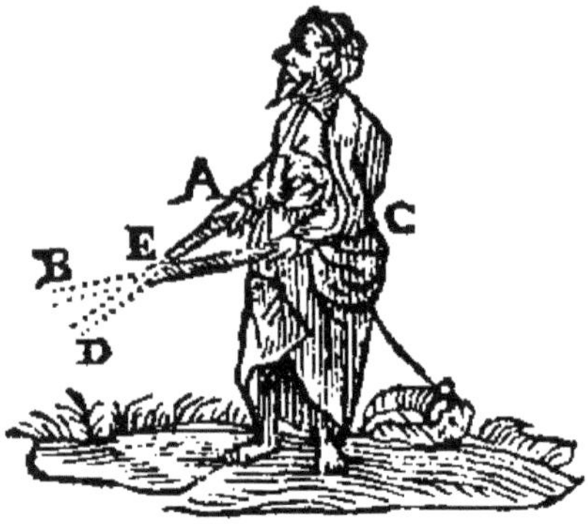

Figure 2 A blind man performing 'natural geometry' from Descartes, *La Dioptrique* (1637).

This second comparison, invoking the same man-born-blind, in the *Dioptrique* serves to explain what he calls 'la géométrie naturelle' [natural geometry],[31] according to which we are able to perceive distance. It appears in both verbal and visual form. The engraving [Figure 2] shows a bearded man, barefoot and dressed like a philosopher in a kind of gown. Given the position of his sticks, he might be taken to be some kind of a water diviner were it not for the presence of the little dog sitting to the right behind him and attached to a leash round his waist, indicating that he is blind.[32] The tufts of grass indicate an outdoor location (perhaps the one described in the earlier analogy), but as the explanatory key (letters A–E) makes clear, he is not so much going for a walk as performing a geometrical calculation: he is triangulating his sticks in order to judge how far away point E is from his hands, which are marked A and C. In fact what the blind man is doing with his sticks is, Descartes explains, what the sighted do all the time without realizing it in the act of visually perceiving spatial distance.[33] As we'll see, this blind man appears in the *Letter*, speaking and giving his explanation of the relationship between touch and sight, and articulating a conception of vision in geometrical terms.

This man-born-blind, who exemplifies a non-representational, anti-Epicurean and geometrical conception of sensory perception, is not the only one to appear in Descartes's writing, however. Moreover, his

31 *Œuvres de Descartes*, vol. 6, p. 136; *The Philosophical Writings of Descartes*, vol. 1, p. 170.

32 It appears twice, see *Œuvres de Descartes*, vol. 6, pp. 135, 136; *The Philosophical Writings of Descartes*, vol. 1, p. 169 (the translation only reproduces it once).

33 The diagram is essentially the same as that representing binocular convergence: the blind man's hands are analogies for the eyes, and his sticks the rays of light touching them.

opponents have a man-born-blind too. And theirs is not an analogy; like Montaigne's gentleman and the men-born-blind of the *Letter*, he is a real person. We find him in Gassendi's objections to Descartes's *Méditations métaphysiques* [Metaphysical Meditations] (1641).

Gassendi's Man-Born-Blind

Descartes's third meditation opens with a declaration signalling that none of the senses is a reliable source of knowledge and that the exemplary case of their unreliability is sight: 'Je fermerai maintenant les yeux' [I will now shut my eyes].[34] To illustrate its unreliability, Descartes explains that the idea of the sun that he gains from his visual experience is tiny, whereas the idea of the sun, which is either innate or produced by geometrical reasoning, is several times larger than the earth. Since it is this latter idea that is accurate, experience can provide no reliable source of knowledge.[35] Such knowledge can only be obtained either from innate ideas or from mathematics, the truths of which are guaranteed by the former, which are themselves guaranteed by God.

To this, Gassendi replies that we simply cannot have any idea of the sun other than the one we gain from our senses. He tells Descartes:

> [V]oulez-vous voir comment la nature n'a rien mis en nous d'une pareille idée? cherchez à la découvrir chez un aveugle-né. Vous verrez d'abord que dans son esprit elle n'est point colorée ou lumineuse; vous verrez ensuite qu'elle n'est point ronde, si quelqu'un ne l'en a averti et s'il n'a lui-même auparavant manié quelque objet rond[.][36]

> If you want to grasp the fact that no part of this idea has been implanted in us by nature, you should inquire about the idea which a man born blind has. You will find first of all that the idea in his mind has no colour or luminosity. Next you will find that it is not even round, unless someone has told him the sun is round and he has previously held a round object in his hands.[37]

The argument from the man-born-blind does not convince Descartes, however, who asks Gassendi to consider why it is that when we close

34 *Œuvres de Descartes*, vol. 9, p. 27; *The Philosophical Writings of Descartes*, vol. 2, p. 24.
35 *Œuvres de Descartes*, vol. 9, p. 31; *The Philosophical Writings of Descartes*, vol. 2, p. 27.
36 Pierre Gassendi, *Disquisitio metaphysica; seu, Dubitationes et instantiae adversus Renati Cartesii Metaphysicam et responsa. Recherches métaphysiques; ou, Doutes et instances contre la Métaphysique de R. Descartes et ses réponses*, Bernard Rochot (ed.) (Paris: Vrin, 1962), p. 226.
37 *The Philosophical Writings of Descartes*, vol. 2, p. 198.

our eyes, we still have some idea of light and colour. He suggests to him that blindness might not be a physical condition in which access to the visual world is blocked, but a mental disorder in which what is lacking in a blind man is not eyes so much as a mind that can see. Descartes says:

> Quand bien même on accorderait ce que vous dites, celui qui nierait l'existence des choses matérielles n'aurait-il pas aussi bien le droit de dire qu'un aveugle-né n'a point d'idées des couleurs parce que son esprit est dépourvu de la faculté de les produire, que vous de dire qu'il ne les a pas parce qu'il est privé d'yeux?[38]

> Even if we grant what you say, those who deny the existence of material things may just as well attribute the absence of ideas of colour in the man-born-blind to the fact that his mind lacks the faculty for forming them; this is just as reasonable as your claim that he does not have the ideas because he is deprived of sight.[39]

In response, a somewhat exasperated Gassendi again refers to a man-born-blind. This time he is not an analogy, nor a conceptual figure, nor an example, but a person whom he once knew:

> J'ai connu autrefois un aveugle de naissance qui travaillait la philosophie sous le même professeur que moi. Je me souviens d'avoir plus d'une fois placé devant lui, tant en plein soleil qu'à l'ombre, diverses couleurs, et de lui avoir dit de se rendre compte s'il y avait quelque différence: or jamais il n'en reconnut aucune. Si vous ne le croyez pas, faites l'expérience.[40]

> I once knew a man who was blind from birth and studied philosophy under the same professor as me. I remember more than once putting various colours before him, in daylight as well as in the shade, and asking him to notice if there was any difference between them, but he never could. If you don't believe it, do the experiment.

Perhaps a real man-born-blind – and a philosopher to boot – will make Descartes see or, rather, make him open his eyes and stop thinking he can see innate ideas in his mind.

Those innate ideas include that of God, as the title of the third meditation suggests: 'De Dieu, qu'il existe' [Of God, that he exists]. Gassendi's man-born-blind is not designed to refute the existence of God, rather

---

38 Descartes in Gassendi, *Disquisitio*, p. 228.
39 *The Philosophical Writings of Descartes*, vol. 2, p. 251.
40 Gassendi, *Disquisitio*, p. 230.

merely to suggest that the purely rationalist nature of Descartes's argument is faulty. However, in the context of an argument in which all ideas come from the senses, an inability to see can easily acquire connotations of religious scepticism, particularly given the powerful presence of images of light and sight in Christian writing. This will be the case in the *Letter*, as we'll see, but it was also suggested in another text about a man-born-blind. This will be the final text in our series. It was written by the sceptical writer and heir to Montaigne, La Mothe Le Vayer.

La Mothe Le Vayer's Man-Born-Blind

'D'un Aveugle-nay' [Of a Man-Born-Blind] is the sixty-fifth of La Mothe Le Vayer's *Petits traités en forme de lettres* [Short Treatises in the Form of Letters] (1653).[41] It takes the form of a paradox, a common form of sceptical, anti-dogmatic writing.[42] It also takes up Gassendi's challenge to Descartes.

It begins by reporting the doxa: sight is the superior sense – philosophy was made visible to man by the gods (Plato); the eye is the noblest of the organs and is to the body what reason is to the soul (Aristotle); visual impressions are more vivid than aural ones (Horace); if some men escaped the Sirens, but none the Gorgons, it was because seeing is faster than hearing (Lucian); the location of the eyes in the human body dictates that of the brain (Galen); and finally, modern science and law both endorse this hierarchy in that the most important recent scientific discoveries come from astronomical observations, and in court, one eye-witness is worth ten aural testimonies. This is a pagan doxa, and it is made up largely of ancient scientific and medical texts as is common in or, rather, is the mark of the writing of the group of freethinking radicals, often known as the 'libertins érudits'.[43] The complete absence of reference to the sacred texts is perhaps more glaring here than elsewhere, given that Christian writing is so full of references to light and sight; their absence suggests the possibility of a sceptical attitude to the Christian revelation.

---

41 See François de La Mothe Le Vayer, *Œuvres*, 7 volumes (Dresden: Michel Groell, 1756), vol. 6, part 2, pp. 123–39. The work is little known today and there is no modern edition. For an English translation, see Appendix Two. Markovits mentions La Mothe Le Vayer's work in passing, see 'L'Aveugle, une figure de la philosophie sceptique', pp. 40, 46.

42 See Rosalie Littell Colie, *Paradoxa Epidemica: The Renaissance Tradition of Paradox* (Princeton: Princeton University Press, 1966); *Heterodoxy in Early Modern Science and Theology*, Ian McLean (ed.) (Oxford: Oxford University Press, 2001), pp. xiv–xx; Agnieszka Steczowicz, *The Defence of Contraries: Paradox in the Late Renaissance Disciplines* (Oxford: D Phil, 2004).

43 The term was invented by René Pintard, see *Le libertinage érudit dans la première moitié du XVIIe siècle*, 2 volumes (Paris: Boivin, 1943). For a recent reappraisal, see Isabelle Moreau, *'Guérir du sot': les stratégies d'écriture des libertins à l'âge classique* (Paris: Champion, 2007).

Before moving on to the para-doxa, the narrator recounts an anecdote, telling of his encounter in Poitiers with a man-born-blind named Dreux La Vallée. Despite the phonetic resemblance between 'La Vallée' and the author's name 'Le Vayer', and despite the fact that both names are close in sound to the verb 'voir' [to see] – a resemblance that La Mothe Le Vayer had in fact already exploited elsewhere in one of his pseudonyms, Orasius, meaning 'little eye'[44] – Dreux La Vallée is neither an imaginary character nor a blind version of the seeing author. He was Jacques Dreux, Seigneur de La Vallée (1604–75), a member of one of the 'good families' of Poitiers and he had probably been blind since birth.[45] His appearance in the text is the tipping point that turns doxa into para-doxa, though it is not itself without dual meaning: it confirms the anti-Cartesian claim that all our knowledge comes from our senses and thus the more senses we have, the more knowledge we have, but it also suggests that seeing is not all it is cracked up to be, and that it may be, as the Epicureans claimed, a species of touch.

Dreux La Vallée is introduced as one of 'les divertissements' [the entertainments] that the narrator enjoyed on his visit to Poitiers, perhaps even as a kind of 'freak show': 'un aveugle né, qu'on m'[. . .] a fait voir' [a man-born-blind whom I have been shown].[46] The relationship is soon presented as more equal, however, as the two men enter into conversation and the narrator informs the reader of La Vallée's background: 'Il est honnête homme, d'une de ces bonnes familles de Poitiers, et qui, nonobstant sa disgrâce, n'a pas laissé d'aller, étant jeune, aux Collèges, et d'y faire des études telles, qu'il a disputé publiquement sur des thèses de philosophie' [He is a gentleman of one of the good families of Poitiers who, despite his misfortune, nonetheless attended the Colleges and advanced far enough with his studies to be able to engage in the public disputation of philosophical theses].[47] This immediately challenges one of the doxical claims which the narrator has just reported, namely that sight is the sense most related to intelligence: here we have a man-born-blind who has been perfectly successful 'despite his misfortune' and, moreover, at philosophy, the discipline most associated with vision. The 'entertainment' that Dreux

44 La Mothe Le Vayer published his *Quatre dialogues faits à l'imitation des Anciens* [Four Dialogues in Imitation of the Ancients] in 1630 under the pseudonym 'Orasius Tubero', and with an invented publisher, place and date of publication (Frankfurt: I. Sarius, 1604). His *Hexaméron rustique* [Rustic Hexameron] appeared in 1670 under the pseudonym 'Tubertu Ocella', where 'ocella' also means 'little eye'.

45 Henri Beauchet-Filleau (ed.), *Dictionnaire historique et généalogique des familles du Poitou* (Poitiers: Oudin, 1891–1979), vol. 3 (1905), p. 16. I am grateful to Eric Puisais for this reference.

46 La Mothe Le Vayer, 'D'un Aveugle-nay', in *Œuvres*, vol. 6, part 2, p. 124; 'Of a Man-Born-Blind', p. 230.

47 La Mothe Le Vayer, *Œuvres*, vol. 6, part 2, p. 128; 'Of a Man-Born-Blind', p. 232.

La Vallée provides is not simply diverting or, rather, it is diverting, but philosophically so, as entertainments so often are in La Mothe Le Vayer.[48]

Their conversation begins with the narrator trying to establish whether his interlocutor really is blind. He says he thought Dreux La Vallée's sight was 'assez nette' [quite clear],[49] akin to that of a sighted man with his eyes closed, and tried to convince him that it was light he could see. Dreux La Vallée explained, however, that he could feel 'un épaississement de l'air' [thickening of the air] and 'la condensation de l'air' [the condensation of the air] which was projected back to him by the objects around him.[50] His vocabulary, also containing terms such as 'prénotion' and 'repercussion', suggests that he has an Epicurean conception of vision, according to which objects emit palpable simulacra.

The narrator agrees, however, that Dreux La Vallée has no idea of colour. Yet, like Montaigne's gentleman, he can talk about them as though he does because, in this case, he has learnt their names and technical terms in his physics lessons. He also has some knowledge of the sun, the subject of such debate between Descartes and Gassendi, and of the moon, the stars, the signs of the zodiac, the tropics, the equinox and the north and south poles, because he has had astronomy lessons, and his teachers allowed him to feel a simulacrum of the globe in his hands.[51] However, the narrator announces, 'avec tout cela il nous pria de croire qu'il ne lui était pas possible de former la moindre conjecture de la beauté de ce grand astre, dont il entendait dire tant de merveilles, ni de tout ce qu'on l'assurait paraître dans les cieux à quiconque pouvait les contempler' [despite all that, he asked us to believe him that it was not possible for him to form the slightest conjecture regarding the beauty of either that big star which he had heard was so marvellous, or of everything which he was told could be seen in the heavens by anyone able to contemplate them].[52] The context is astronomy, but terms like 'beauty' and 'marvellous' gesture towards natural theology and the argument for God's existence on the basis of the visible evidence in nature – evidence that is, of course, not available to the blind man.

Nothing is made in La Mothe Le Vayer's 'opuscule' [little work] of the sceptical possibilities of the blind man's inability to see the beauty and marvel of the world, however. Instead, the narrator proposes a generic conclusion to his story: it was a philosophical fable, illustrating the Aristotelian maxim: 'Vous voyez en tout cela clairement la preuve de

48 See Sylvia Giocanti, 'La Mothe Le Vayer: modes de diversion sceptique'. *Libertinage et philosophie au XVIIe siècle*, 2 (1997), 33–48, 33.
49 La Mothe Le Vayer, *Œuvres*, vol. 6, part 2, p. 128; 'Of a Man-Born-Blind', p. 232.
50 La Mothe Le Vayer, *Œuvres*, vol. 6, part 2, p. 129; 'Of a Man-Born-Blind', p. 232.
51 La Mothe Le Vayer, *Œuvres*, vol. 6, part 2, pp. 130–1; 'Of a Man-Born-Blind', p. 232.
52 La Mothe Le Vayer, *Œuvres*, vol. 6, part 2, p. 131; 'Of a Man-Born-Blind', p. 232.

l'axiome philosophique, qu'il n'entre rien dans notre esprit que par la porte des sens; et par conséquent, que si l'on manque de quelqu'un, notre âme est nécessairement privée de beaucoup de connaissances' [In all this, you can see clear proof of the philosophical axiom, according to which nothing enters our minds except through the senses, and consequently, if we are lacking in one sense, our soul is necessarily deprived of much knowledge].[53] So the diverting conversation with Dreux La Vallée has proved that Gassendi's objection to Descartes was right, because his lack of sight does indeed deny him access to ideas such as colour and beauty. Moreover, in both cases, it was a philosopher-born-blind who did so.[54]

The text does not end on this note, however. Though blindness does block access to ideas, the narrator turns the conclusion back on itself, relating the para-doxa according to which sight is a sense we could well do without. He explains that it prevents the other senses from working properly, which is why we close our eyes to listen to music or to savour a taste. History contains many remarkable blind men who saw more clearly precisely because they were blind (Appius Claudius, Democritus, Homer, Tiresias), and sight causes more pain than pleasure (Ovid was exiled for seeing something he wasn't supposed to; the city is full of ugliness; it is not necessarily desirable to be looked at). And so, paradoxical to the very last, La Mothe Le Vayer's little work concludes as follows:

> Bref, à moins que de tomber dans un aveuglement d'esprit, on ne doutera jamais des désavantages que cause celui du corps. Mais, tournez la médaille, vous verrez, qu'on n'en évite pas d'autres encore plus grands, pour avoir bonne vue, et si vous serez contraints de confesser, que la cécité a ses biens et ses privilèges encore plus grands que nous ne les avons remarqués, ne fût-ce que quand nous cédons le haut du pavé aux aveugles comme aux plus grands seigneurs. Pour conclusion permettez-moi cette petite raillerie en faveur des premiers, que si le texte d'Aristote est véritable, qu'aux pourceaux la perte d'un œil est la perte de la vie, on peut dire que c'est tenir plus du pourceaux que de l'homme raisonnable, de ne pouvoir vivre sans yeux.[55]

> In short, unless we succumb to mental blindness, we shall never underestimate the disadvantages of physical blindness. But on the

53 La Mothe Le Vayer, *Œuvres*, vol. 6, part 2, p. 131; 'Of a Man-Born-Blind', p. 232.

54 La Mothe Le Vayer may be drawing on other paradoxical texts such as Ortensio Landi's *Paradossi* [Paradoxes] (1543), which was translated into French by Charles Estienne in 1553/4. See Estienne, *Paradoxes*, Trevor Peach (ed.) (Geneva: Droz, 1998) and Steczowicz, *The Defence of Contraries*.

55 La Mothe Le Vayer, *Œuvres*, vol. 6, part 2, p. 139.

> other hand, you will see that greater disadvantages are not avoided by being able to see, and you will have to admit that blindness has its advantages and privileges, some of which are even greater than those we have observed so far, not least that we step into the gutter for the blind, as we do for the greatest noblemen. In conclusion, allow me this little mockery in favour of the former, and let me say that if Aristotle's text is correct and for pigs, losing an eye means losing their life, it may be said that we would be more like pigs than reasonable men, if we could not live without eyes.[56]

It is with these men-born-blind in mind – be they examples, analogies or real people, be they, in turn, aristocrats, fools or philosophers – that we return to the *Letter*.

---

56 La Mothe Le Vayer, 'Of a Man-Born-Blind', p. 237.

Three

Point of View and *Point de Vue*

What are the man-born-blind-of-Puiseaux's views on morals and metaphysics? In raising this question, the *Letter* exploits in multiple ways the self-reflexive possibilities involved in the sighted observing the blind and seeing that they are blind too – not for nothing are mirrors one of the topics of the reported conversation with the man-born-blind of Puiseaux. That conversation and ***'s presentation of it, which are the focus of this chapter, explore a range of topics and make a number of moves that replay and rework what Montaigne, Descartes, Gassendi and La Mothe Le Vayer said about men-born-blind, as well as what their men-born-blind themselves said. And one of the things that emerges is captured by the French phrase 'point de vue', namely that 'point of view', because it is itself always the object of another's, is 'point de vue', that is, blind.[1] The moves the text makes in this section are not all reciprocal and self-reflexive, however; the discussions of morals and metaphysics also involve some much less symmetrical relationships, and it is in this part of the *Letter* that some of ***'s most arresting and paradoxical claims are to be found.

Reflections and Refractions

The story of *** and his friends' visit to Puiseaux has much in common with the epistolary travel narratives that were popular in eighteenth-century fiction, such as Montesquieu's *Lettres persanes* [Persian Letters] (1721), Voltaire's *Lettres philosophiques* [Letters on the English Nation] (1733/4) and Graffigny's *Lettres d'une Péruvienne* [Letters from a Peruvian Woman] (1747, second edition 1752), all of which owe much to Montaigne's essay, 'Des cannibales' [Of Cannibals]. Indeed, in this sense, the *Letter* seems to have more in common with Foucault's other foundational myth of the

---

1 Interplay of gazes is a frequent theme in Diderot's later writing. Hobson has observed, for example, the strange reciprocity envisaged in the claim made in the *Commentaire sur Hemsterhuis* [Commentary on Hemsterhuis] (1773–4): 'l'œil ne voit strictement que le point qui le fixe' [the eye only strictly sees the point that is staring at it] (quoted in *Diderot and Rousseau*, p. 89). It is curious that this interplay has not been studied in the *Letter*, in which it is not only an obvious theme but also a defining feature of the writing.

Enlightenment, namely the foreign spectator in an unknown land.[2]

***'s narrative begins with some scene setting in which we are told, for example, that *** and his friends arrived at the man-born-blind-of-Puiseaux's house at five o'clock in the evening to find him not long out of bed and teaching his son to read using raised characters. Keen to find out what the man-born-blind knows about sight and visual phenomena, the visitors ask him what he thinks mirrors and eyesight are. He replies with what appear to be Cartesian definitions that provoke admiration and wonder. These are the first instances of an emotion that is presented throughout the *Letter* in highly ambivalent ways. In this case, it is an important aspect of the presentation of Cartesian science in the *Letter*, which is sufficiently ambiguous to have prompted entirely divergent opinions as to its status in the text. For Jessica Riskin, the *Letter* presents Cartesianism as being without merit;[3] for Véronique Le Ru and for André Charrak, by contrast, it can be read as promoting many aspects of Descartes's method and discoveries.[4]

The man-born-blind of Puiseaux defined a mirror as follows: 'Une machine [. . .] qui met les choses en relief, loin d'elles-mêmes, si elles se trouvent placées convenablement par rapport à elle. C'est comme ma main qu'il ne faut pas que je pose à côté d'un objet pour le sentir' [A machine [. . .] that projects things in three dimensions at a distance from themselves, if they are correctly placed in front of it. It is like my hand inasmuch as I mustn't place it to one side of an object if I want to feel it].[5] And *** comments, 'Descartes aveugle-né, aurait dû, ce me semble, s'applaudir d'une pareille définition.' [Had Descartes been born blind, he would, it seems to me, have congratulated himself on such a definition].[6] There are a number of most peculiar aspects to this definition and the commentary.

The blind man's definition of a mirror is enlightening with respect to his analogical mode of thinking that translates the catoptrical qualities of the mirror into terms related to touch. However, it is not very enlightening with respect to the nature of a mirror. In fact, this is underlined in the second sentence of the definition that refers to a situation in which reflection is impossible because the necessary conditions have not been

---

2 Foucault, *Birth of the Clinic*, p. 65.

3 Jessica Riskin, *Science in the Age of Sensibility* (Chicago: University of Chicago Press, 2002), pp. 21–2, 61–2.

4 Véronique Le Ru, 'La *Lettre sur les aveugles* et le bâton de la raison'. *Recherches sur Diderot et l'Encyclopédie*, 28 (2000), 25–41; André Charrak, 'Géométrie et métaphysique dans la *Lettre sur les aveugles* de Diderot'. *Recherches sur Diderot et l'Encyclopédie*, 28 (2000), 43–53.

5 DPV, 4, p. 20; Hobson and Harvey, p. 31; *Letter*, p. 173.

6 DPV, 4, p. 20; Hobson and Harvey, p. 31; *Letter*, p. 173.

met.[7] Moreover, the comparison, 'It's like my hand', introduces as much difference between seeing and touching as it does similarity: as the man-born-blind's terms 'at a distance' and 'not . . . to one side' make clear, while hands and mirrors do have to be 'suitably positioned' with respect to the object we want them to reflect, a mirror requires the object to be placed at a distance, which is precisely the opposite of that required by the hand, namely proximity, which enables it to feel the object.

As for ***'s commentary referring to Descartes, it confirms that something strange is going on. The blind man's definition sounds as Aristotelian or Epicurean as it does Cartesian – in *De Rerum Natura*, Lucretius speaks of the mirror image as an appearance 'flung straight back / In reverse, as if someone should throw a mask / Of plaster before it is dry against a pillar / So that it bounces straight back keeping the features / Set on its front, but showing them in reverse'.[8] And moreover, the praise for the blind man's definition of the mirror image by analogy with a palpable object is not voiced by *** (still less by Diderot), but by Descartes or, more precisely, an imaginary, congenitally blind Descartes. Praise is undermined by so many levels of mediation. Furthermore, the imaginary blind Descartes does not so much congratulate the blind man on his definition as congratulate himself on his own – he even does so using his hands: 'applaudir', used here reflexively, means 'to clap'. This is no straightforward endorsement of Cartesian science.

If the exchange between *** and the man-born-blind of Puiseaux concentrates on mirrors, it is because their effect is to make touch and sight contradict each other. The mirror image is imperceptible to the blind man; it lies beyond his grasp and is therefore an object of wonder and admiration to him.[9] Showing off their greater knowledge, *** and his friends take pleasure in recounting what for him are fantastical tales of optical instruments – not only mirrors, but telescopes and microscopes too – all of which alter the object visually in a manner that astounds the blind man who, unable to understand what they are talking about, asks hundreds of 'bizarre' questions. Here, however, as elsewhere in the *Letter*, as we'll see, the blind man of Puiseaux is not to be outdone, and he comes

---

7 The same is true of the second part of his definition of eyesight, which also refers to a hand obstructing vision, see DPV, 4, p. 21; Hobson and Harvey, p. 33; *Letter*, p. 174.

8 Lucretius, *On the Nature of the Universe*, Ronald Melville (trans.) Don and Peta Fowler (intro. and notes) (Oxford: Oxford World's Classics, 1997), p. 109 (Book IV, lines 295–9). The 'Apology' also draws on and explicitly quotes Lucretius. See *Essais*, p. 592; *Essays*, pp. 542–3. For Aristotle on touch, see Daniel Heller-Roazen, *The Inner Touch: Archeology of a Sensation* (Cambridge, MA: MIT Press, 2007).

9 Mirrors are a classic topos of travel narratives. See, for instance, Françoise de Graffigny, *Lettres d'une Péruvienne*, Jonathan Mallinson (ed.) (Oxford: Voltaire Foundation, 2002), p. 134.

up with some dazzling inventions of his own: he describes a machine that would override the contradictions between sight and touch or, better still, that would make sensory perceptions disappear altogether and notify us of our mistake. Inasmuch as this latter machine is designed to bring touch and sight into line with the aim of banishing error, it sounds rather like Cartesian metaphysics; indeed no sooner has he finished describing it than we are shown what it might look like: the *Letter* reproduces the engraving from Descartes's *Dioptrique* of the blind man holding two crossed sticks (see the first plate of the *Letter*, p. 175). The man-born-blind of Puiseaux seems to have been envisaging the Cartesian geometrization of vision.

This too is open to dual interpretation. The engraving reproduced in the *Letter* is not identical to Descartes' original and the differences are worth emphasising. Whereas Descartes's diagram showed an old, bearded, shabbily dressed blind man, surrounded by an explanatory key, the *Letter* shows a drawing of a young, clean-shaven, well-dressed young man wearing a blindfold. This picture is taken from an eighteenth-century edition of *La Dioptrique*,[10] and yet there is a sense in which the science of optics has been turned into a fashionable parlour game – a kind of blind man's buff with sticks. Moreover, as though seen in a mirror, the figure has been reversed: in the *Discours*, he looks to the left, in the *Letter*, to the right.

Moreover, ***'s commentary is highly ambiguous. He says: 'Descartes et tous ceux qui sont venus depuis, n'ont pu nous donner d'idées plus nettes de la vision; et ce grand philosophe n'a point eu à cet égard plus d'avantage sur notre aveugle, que le peuple qui a des yeux' [Descartes and all those who have come after him have been unable to provide any clearer ideas of vision, and in this respect, the great philosopher's superiority over our blind man was no greater than that of the common man, who can see].[11] On the one hand, Cartesian theory, which conceives of vision blindly – that is, in geometrical terms – is the best theory we have and, as we'll see, it allowed Saunderson to lecture successfully on optics.[12] On the other hand, Descartes' analogy is turned against him – his theory of vision is no better than that of a blind man, to whom he is only superior by virtue of his sight, which he shares with the man in the street.

As observed earlier, Riskin has read the *Letter*'s presentation of Cartesian science as unambiguously negative. In addition, she claims that the *Letter* condemns Cartesians and the blind on grounds that are not only scientific, but also moral. Her reading of the men-born-blind in

---

10 It is taken from René Descartes, *Discours de la méthode* (Paris: Nicolas Poisson, 1724).
11 DPV, 4, p. 21; Hobson and Harvey, p. 33; *Letter*, p. 174.
12 DPV, 4, p. 42; Hobson and Harvey, p. 54; *Letter*, p. 194.

the *Letter* as morally and visually challenged has been influential,[13] and so it requires examination.

Morally Blind?

The man-born-blind of Puiseaux is fond of order and symmetry, and he likes to keep his house tidy so that he can find things easily. In a move calculated to make Madame fond of the man-born-blind, *** tells her, 'quand sa femme s'éveille, elle trouve ordinairement la maison rangée' [his wife usually wakes up to a tidy house].[14] Living with a blind man has other benefits too – moral ones as well as ones related to domestic comforts: it makes the sighted less untidy and more compassionate 'soit par un effet du bon exemple qu'ils donnent, soit par un sentiment d'humanité qu'on a pour eux' [either owing to their good example or out of a feeling of empathy that we have for them].[15] This is the beginning of a thread that runs throughout the *Letter* concerning the relative humanity of the blind and the sighted, and the idea of the human as a relative moral category.[16]

The compassion of the sighted for the blind prompts *** to utter a condescending exclamation: 'Que les aveugles seraient malheureux sans les petites attentions de ceux qui les environnent!' [How unhappy the blind would be without the small acts of kindness of those around them!][17] Such a position of superiority with regard to the poor blind is immediately undercut, however, by a second more self-reflexive exclamation: 'Nous-mêmes, que nous serions à plaindre sans elles!' [And how unhappy we would be too!].[18] The sighted, it turns out, are no less dependent on the kindness of other people than the blind, and moreover, as we'll see, exclamation is a mode of utterance that is often treated ironically in the *Letter*. The reciprocal – tidy and symmetrical – relationship suggested here does not come to a completely stable resting place, however, for when one of the central terms, 'humanité' [empathy], is mentioned a little later, the relationship between the blind and the sighted shifts again.

If the sighted perform little acts of kindness for the blind, such acts, without which the sighted would be just as unhappy as the blind, are not performed by the blind for the sighted. The sighted are the objects

---

13 See Stephen Gaukroger, ''Home Alone': Cognitive Solipsism in the Early-Modern Era'. *Proceedings and Addresses of the American Philosophical Association*, 80.2 (2006), 63–78.

14 DPV, 4, p. 19; Hobson and Harvey, p. 30; *Letter*, p. 172.

15 DPV, 4, p. 19; Hobson and Harvey, p. 30; *Letter*, p. 172.

16 For a study of the evolution of the terms 'human' and 'inhuman' in the period, which also makes brief reference to the ideas of the *Letter*, see James A. Steintrager, *Cruel Delight: Enlightenment Culture and the Inhuman* (Bloomington: Indiana University Press, 2004), pp. 79–80.

17 DPV, 4, p. 19; Hobson and Harvey, p. 30; *Letter*, p. 172.

18 DPV, 4, p. 19; Hobson and Harvey, p. 30; *Letter*, p. 172.

of kindness only on the part of other sighted people, because the blind are unable to perceive the suffering of others which is, according to ***, expressed primarily visually. As a result, he says, 'je les soupçonne en général d'inhumanité.' [I suspect them, in general, of being inhumane].[19] Moreover, hearing is not reliable when it comes to sensing others' pain as some things sound the same: 'Quelle différence y a-t-il pour un aveugle entre un homme qui urine et un homme qui sans se plaindre verse son sang?' [What difference can there be for a blind man between a man urinating and a man shedding blood without a whimper?].[20]

This rather disturbing question provoked a defensive response from a blind acquaintance of Diderot – Mélanie de Salignac – which he included in the later 'Additions'; and critics have sought to defend Diderot: Riskin has interpreted it as an indictment of a Cartesian rationalist disregard for sensory evidence, which she claims is presented in the *Letter* as selfish, even solipsistic.[21] Certainly in retrospect, as we'll see, the question of the blind's failure to be compassionate will acquire philosophical implications, though not quite the ones Riskin has put forward. However, ***'s outlandish comparison between urinating and bleeding is here designed to expose the much more banal acts of inhumanity that are committed by the sighted, as the *Letter* gives a moral twist to the numerous contemporary debates over the perception of size and distance that are to be found in optical and epistemological theory of the period. These sought to explain how we understand that a distant object, though it appears tiny, is in reality not so. *** suggests that since the visual perception of size varies according to distance, there can be no absolute values in the sighted moral code. He asks, 'Nous-mêmes, ne cessons-nous pas de compatir, lorsque la distance ou la petitesse des objets produit le même effet sur nous, que la privation de la vue sur les aveugles?' [Don't we too stop sympathising when something is so far away or so small that we can't see it any more clearly than a blind man can?],[22] and observes that we squash ants and, 'sans la crainte du châtiment' [were it not for fear of punishment],[23] many would rather shoot a man at a distance than kill a bull with their bare hands. The blind may be inhumane, but they can't help it; the sighted, on the other hand, should know better.

Fear of punishment is key and the blind are, it seems, immune to it.

19 DPV, 4, p. 27; Hobson and Harvey, p. 38; *Letter*, p. 38.

20 DPV, 4, p. 27; Hobson and Harvey, p. 38; *Letter*, p. 38.

21 Riskin asserts: 'Diderot gave his moral repudiation of Cartesianism a literal, physiological meaning in the [*Letter*]. Cartesians thought like blind men, and the blind were inhumane. The conclusion was plain to see' (*Science in an Age of Sensibility*, p. 61; see also pp. 11, 21–2).

22 DPV, 4, p. 27; Hobson and Harvey, p. 38; *Letter*, p. 38.

23 DPV, 4, p. 27; Hobson and Harvey, p. 38; *Letter*, p. 38.

*** recounts an anecdote that recalls Montaigne's hunting and shooting blind gentleman though, unlike his predecessor, the man-born-blind of Puiseaux is an excellent shot (and doesn't have servants to tell him where to aim). In fact, he's so accurate that he's dangerous: in anger, he once threw something at his brother and knocked him out cold. The matter went to court, where not only did the visible signs of the judge's authority not intimidate the blind man, but when the judge threatened to punish him by throwing him in the dungeon, he quipped, 'Eh, Monsieur [. . .] il y a vingt-cinq ans que j'y suis' [Oh Sir [. . .] That's where I've been for twenty-five years].[24] The blind are, it seems, not only in general inhumane, but they are also incorrigible by the normal, that is to say, sighted means. It is also hinted that the man-born-blind is a man-born-condemned, and the question of the justice meted out by a judge who is greater in power than the court magistrate is one to which the *Letter* will return.

Other aspects of the man-born-blind-of-Puiseaux's behaviour recall that of the comic type: the thief and the lecher. We are initially told, and it would seem to fit with his difficulty in finding things in the house when they are not where he thought they were, that the man-born-blind of Puiseaux finds theft particularly abhorrent. *** explains that it is owing to 'la facilité qu'on avait de le voler, sans qu'il s'en aperçût' [the ease with which other people could steal from him without him noticing]. We are then surprised to discover that his abhorrence for theft is the greater owing to '[la facilité] qu'on avait de l'apercevoir, quand il volait' [[the ease] with which they could see him stealing from them].[25] The blind man is as much a perpetrator of theft as a victim of it. Moreover, in a highly disconcerting move, *** reports, 'Ce n'est pas qu'il ne sache très bien se mettre en garde contre le sens qu'il nous connaît de plus qu'à lui, et qu'il ignore la manière de bien cacher un vol' [It's not that he doesn't know perfectly well how to guard himself against the additional sense he knows us to have, nor that he is unaware of how best to cover up a theft].[26] *** refuses to divulge here what the thieving blind man's tactics are for evading our gaze and thereby raises an uneasy sense in the reader that he is in cahoots with the blind – *** might be hoodwinking us too.

*** suggests that the man-born-blind of Puiseaux may not be averse to turning his disability to his advantage. Reporting on his excellent sense of touch as well as hearing, *** imagines the standard comic gag: '[l]e poli des corps n'a guère moins de nuances pour lui, que le son de la voix; et il n'y aurait pas à craindre qu'il prît sa femme pour une autre, à moins qu'il ne gagnât au change' [The surface of the skin is no less subtly differentiated to him than the sound of the voice, and there is no reason to

24 DPV, 4, p. 24; Hobson and Harvey, p. 35; *Letter*, p. 177.
25 DPV, 4, pp. 26–7; Hobson and Harvey, pp. 37–8; *Letter*, p. 179.
26 DPV, 4, pp. 26–7; Hobson and Harvey, pp. 37–8; *Letter*, p. 179.

fear he might mistake his wife for another woman, unless he stood to gain by it].[27] Yet he can also himself be easily deceived, and *** reports that, in a land of the blind, either wives would have to be held in common or adultery laws would have to be particularly severe because 'Il serait si facile aux femmes de tromper leurs maris, en convenant d'un signe avec leurs amants' [It would be very easy for wives to deceive their husbands by using a sign they had agreed with their lovers].[28] The complicity is now between *** and those who deceive the blind, and the reference to wives cheating on blind husbands is a classic topos of libertine painting: the spectator of Greuze's *L'Aveugle trompé* [The Blind Man Deceived] (1755), for instance, takes pleasure in observing an old blind man being unable to see his young wife making a sign to her lover.[29]

This is pure speculation on ***'s part, combined with a dose of voyeurism, and it comes to an end when we hear what the man-born-blind himself thinks. *** reports that the man-born-blind told him that if it weren't for the protection clothes afforded from draughts, he couldn't see the point of wearing them, particularly the sort that prevents one part of the body from expressing itself freely. *** is quick to say to his female correspondent that he doesn't endorse the blind man's failure to grasp modesty and rather grandly asserts:

> Quoique nous soyons dans un siècle où l'esprit philosophique nous a débarrassé d'un grand nombre de préjugés, je ne crois pas que nous en venions jamais jusqu'à méconnaître les prérogatives de la pudeur aussi parfaitement que mon aveugle. Diogène n'aurait point été pour lui un philosophe.[30]
>
> Although we live in a century in which the philosophical spirit has rid us of a great number of prejudices, I don't think we will ever go so far as to misunderstand the obligations of modesty quite as completely as my blind man. To him, Diogenes would not have been a philosopher.[31]

That final claim is rather sudden and gives pause for thought: Diogenes' nakedness and lewd behaviour was a constant affront to public decency because it was visible. In a land of the blind, Diogenes would have to find

27 DPV, 4, p. 24; Hobson and Harvey, p. 36; *Letter*, p. 177.
28 DPV, 4, pp. 24–5; Hobson and Harvey, p. 36; *Letter*, p. 177. The phrase 'land of the blind' is ambiguous: it's not clear whether it refers only to the male inhabitants or whether the wives are blind too.
29 The painting is held in the Pushkin Fine Arts Museum, Moscow.
30 DPV, 4, p. 27; Hobson and Harvey, p. 38.
31 *Letter*, p. 179.

non-visual ways of upsetting social customs (perhaps he could contrive to have no sense of 'personal space'). Yet while it is possible to imagine a Diogenes for the blind, that isn't quite what ***'s statement is suggesting; the blind man wouldn't have thought Diogenes was a philosopher, but might we take the blind man to be one? The outsider position of the man-born-blind in the land of the sighted allows him to point out that moral values are relative, in this case, to our bodily organisation; modesty is a purely sighted value. In a land of the blind, bodies could express themselves freely, and that suggestion of freedom of the body prepares the way for what will be Saunderson's freedom of thought and verbal expression.

The *Letter* ensures then that the sighted reader cannot comfortably feel superior to the blind, either philosophically or morally, and, as in Montaigne, there are frequent suggestions that the sighted are no less blind than the blind. But might the blind be in some sense superior to the sighted? This has often been taken to be the central message of the *Letter* and that may be right but, as we'll see, it is nonetheless presented in some highly unstable ways.

Blind Vanity

*** reports that the man-born-blind had a firm view on the question of the relative merits of blindness and sight: he says that 'il se trouverait fort à plaindre d'être privé des mêmes avantages que nous, et qu'il aurait été tenté de nous regarder comme des intelligences supérieures, s'il n'avait éprouvé cent fois, combien nous lui cédions à d'autres égards' [he might have thought himself to be pitied for lacking our advantages and might have been tempted to see us as superior beings, had he not on hundreds of occasions felt how much we deferred to him in other ways].[32] This prompts a quite spectacular reaction in ***, which is worth quoting in full:

> Cet aveugle, dîmes-nous, s'estime autant et plus peut-être que nous qui voyons; pourquoi donc si l'animal raisonne, comme on n'en peut guère douter, balançant ses avantages sur l'homme, qui lui sont mieux connus que ceux de l'homme sur lui, ne porterait-il pas un semblable jugement? Il a des bras, dit peut-être le moucheron; mais j'ai des ailes. S'il a des armes, dit le lion, n'avons-nous pas des ongles? L'éléphant nous verra comme des insectes; et tous les animaux, nous accordant volontiers une raison avec laquelle nous aurions grand besoin de leur instinct, se prétendront doués d'un instinct avec lequel ils se passent fort bien de notre raison. Nous avons un si violent penchant à surfaire nos qualités et à diminuer

32 DPV, 4, p. 23; Hobson and Harvey, p. 34; *Letter*, p. 176.

nos défauts, qu'il semblerait presque, que c'est à l'homme à faire le traité de la force, et à l'animal, celui de la raison.[33]

This blind man, we said to ourselves, has as high a regard for himself as he does for those of us who can see, perhaps higher; why then if an animal has reason, which we can hardly doubt, and if it weighed up its advantages over those of man, which it knows better than man's over it, would it not pass a similar judgement? He has arms, the fly might say, but I have wings. Though he has weapons, says the lion, do we not have claws? The elephant will see us as insects; and while all animals are happy to grant us our reason, which leaves us in great need of their instinct, they claim to be possessed of an instinct, which gives them no need for our reason. We have such a strong tendency to overstate our qualities and underplay our faults that it would almost seem as though man should be the one to do the treatise on strength and animals the one on reason.[34]

The relativizing comparison between animals and humans is a classic topos of the sceptical tradition – indeed we met it earlier with La Mothe Le Vayer's pig. But it is rather peculiar here, not least because humans and animals do not map in any stable ways onto sighted and blind, and point of view is particularly mobile. The sighted imagine the blind man's point of view on himself in relation to sighted ('[t]his blind man, we said to ourselves'); that point of view then becomes that of the animals as the sighted imagine how the animals view themselves in relation to humans ('[h]e has arms, the fly might say'); and finally the sighted use the first-person plural pronoun, 'we', to voice the point of view of all humans and all animals on themselves in relation to each other, revealing it – blind, sighted, human, animal, insect, mammalian – to be vain ('[w]e have such a strong tendency to overstate our qualities') and therefore, metaphorically, blind.

We should not be blinded, however, by that final neat moralising chiasmus. ***'s appeal to the entire human and animal kingdom in order to re-establish equal relations between the sighted and the blind suggests his sighted pride has been injured, Moreover, the neatness of morality suggests that it is a kind of official discourse, designed to contain the implications of the blind man's challenge to the sighted that is masquerading as the animal challenge to the human. Moreover, on close inspection, it only appears to re-establish an equilibrium: if *** begins by 'hardly doubt[ing]' that animals can reason, he goes on to claim that they have

33 DPV, 4, p. 23; Hobson and Harvey, pp. 34–5.
34 *Letter*, p. 176.

no need for reason since they have animal instinct, which we lack. ***'s claim is subtly loaded against his own side.

We might wonder, of course, what side *** is really on. Indeed, here the moralizing high ground does not silence the man-born-blind of Puiseaux or, rather, it does not prevent *** from continuing to report his views: asked if he would like to see, he replied he'd rather have longer arms because touch has no vanishing point and hands do not, as it were, lose their touch. And *** goes on to provides many examples of the blind man's superior abilities, such as his judgement of the passing of time, his greater sensitivity to weights and measures, and to his wife's skin.[35]

At one point in the *Letter*, the blind man is heard to voice irritation at *** and his friends, owing to their constant and patronizing expression of wonder at his abilities. He quips, 'je m'aperçois bien, Messieurs, [. . .] que vous n'êtes pas aveugles: vous êtes surpris de ce que je fais, et pourquoi ne vous étonnez-vous pas aussi de ce que je parle?' [it is clear to me, Gentlemen, [. . .] that you are not blind since you are surprised at what I can do. So why aren't you also amazed that I can speak?].[36] His relationship to language and how it differs from that of the sighted person is a recurrent and important theme throughout the text.

Optics and Phatics

The nature of the relationship between words and ideas in mind was much discussed in the period – Book Four of Locke's *Essay* is entirely devoted to language or what he calls 'words', as is the whole of the second part of Condillac's *Essai*. There are, however, significant differences between the set of remarks about language in the *Letter* and early modern and Enlightenment linguistic theory. The latter usually examines the relationship between words and ideas with the aim of eradicating a blind or referent-free use of language, deemed to be the source of much confusion. For Locke, scholastic terminology is lacking in referents, and extra care must be taken when using words such as 'justice' or 'beauty' that refer to complex ideas and are thereby more easily misapplied than words referring to simple ideas like 'red' or 'hot'. The *Letter*, by contrast, is more ambivalent, constantly and amusingly drawing our attention to the blind man's blind use of language, which produces surprisingly successful communication.

*** is initially unchastized by the blind man's quip about his ability to speak, saying that it is indeed surprising: 'Il y a, je crois, plus de philosophie dans cette réponse qu'il ne prétendait y en mettre lui-même' [There is, I believe, more philosophy in that reply than he intended].[37] He goes

35 DPV, 4, p. 24; Hobson and Harvey, p. 35–6; *Letter*, p. 177.
36 DPV, 4, p. 25; Hobson and Harvey, p. 37; *Letter*, p. 178.
37 DPV, 4, p. 25–6; Hobson and Harvey, p. 37; *Letter*, p. 178.

on to explain in Lockean terms how ideas must be attached to words and how this is more difficult for a blind man than for the sighted because he has fewer ideas. However, his example of the word 'physiognomy' rather undercuts his explanation: '[c]'est une espèce d'agrément qui consiste en des objets si peu sensibles pour un aveugle, que faute de l'être assez pour nous-mêmes qui voyons, nous serions fort embarrassés de dire bien précisément ce que c'est que d'avoir de la physionomie' [It is a charming kind of quality consisting of things that are so barely perceptible to a blind man and hardly more so to those of us who can see, that we would have great trouble saying exactly what it is to be possessed of a physiognomy].[38] Our idea of what it is is barely any better than a blind man's, and most of ***'s examples have this reflexive effect.

He reports that although the the man-born-blind can't see beauty, he makes use of words such as 'beautiful' that have a visual referent: 'quand il dit, *cela est beau*, il ne juge pas, il rapporte seulement le jugement de ceux qui voient: et que font autre chose les trois quarts de ceux qui décident d'une pièce de théâtre, après l'avoir entendue, ou d'un livre, après l'avoir lu?' [when he says *that's beautiful*, he is not judging it to be so, he is simply repeating the judgement of the sighted. And is that any different to what three quarters of people do when they judge a play they have listened to or a book they have read?].[39] This brings out all the more explicitly what Montaigne also suggested, namely that language works perfectly well referent-blind; its function is often phatic. In this case, however, ***'s commentary might better be described as refractive than reflexive. He is not saying that when it comes to beauty, everyone is blind – some people do have an idea of beauty, namely the remaining one quarter of theatre-goers. Instead, what he is saying is that if the blind don't know what beauty is, they're not the only ones. This leaves a space – what we might think of as a blind spot (or perhaps a sighted spot in the blind mirror) – in which we might find people who do not simply repeat what other people say. That space may be quite small, but it might be significant, and certainly we should look out – or listen out – for it.

*** even goes so far as to suggest that perceptual access to a referent might even act as an impediment to successful communication or, at least, that it might lead speakers to use words in inappropriate ways. Although the man-born-blind of Puiseaux lacks a perceptual referent for the term 'mirror' or, rather, is unable to perceive its specific catoptric qualities (he can of course feel other qualities), this seems to have no effect on his ability to place either the object or the term correctly. Indeed, in the latter case, it seems to make him better at doing so: 's'il n'attache aucune idée

38 DPV, 4, p. 26; Hobson and Harvey, p. 37; *Letter*, p. 178.
39 DPV, 4, p. 19; Hobson and Harvey, p. 30; *Letter*, p. 172.

aux termes qu'il emploie, il a du moins sur la plupart des autres hommes l'avantage de ne les prononcer jamais mal à propos' [though he does not attach any ideas to the terms he uses, he nonetheless has an advantage over most other men in that he never uses them incorrectly].[40] It sounds as though the blind man's ability to say the right thing at the right time depends on his speech being free of referential content. If you know he is blind, his use of language seems, as Montaigne put it, 'private', or, rather, as *** observes, it suggests that what is going on 'inside him' is quite different from what is going on inside us: 'Il discourt si bien et si juste de tant de choses qui lui sont absolument inconnues, que son commerce ôterait beaucoup de force à cette induction que nous faisons tous, sans savoir pourquoi, de ce qui se passe en nous, à ce qui se passe au dedans des autres' [He speaks so well and so accurately on so many things that are absolutely unknown to him, that conversing with him would undermine the inductive reasoning we all perform, though we have no idea why, which assumes that what goes on inside us is the same as what goes on inside others].[41] If, on the other hand, you didn't know he was blind and were to listen to the man-born-blind of Puiseaux talk about mirrors, there'd be no way of knowing he was. Here the most disconcerting thing about the blind is not that they are different to the sighted, but that they sound exactly the same.

The epigraph has been inverted here: 'they can, though they don't look as though they can' has become 'they can't, but they sound as though they can'. Not for long, however, as *** goes on to examine the sceptical implications, already evoked by La Mothe Le Vayer, of the inability of the blind to see the marvels of nature.

Blind Metaphysics

Having just observed that 'our' metaphysics is no more in agreement with 'theirs' than 'our' morality – a comparison that subtly positions the blind in the position of the orthodox – *** says:

> Je pourrais entrer là-dessus dans un détail qui vous amuserait sans doute, mais que de certaines gens qui voient du crime à tout, ne manqueraient pas d'accuser d'irréligion, comme s'il dépendait de moi de faire apercevoir aux aveugles, les choses autrement qu'ils ne les aperçoivent.[42]

> I could go into detail about that here, which would no doubt be to your amusement, but some people who see crime everywhere

40 DPV, 4, p. 20; Hobson and Harvey, p. 31; *Letter*, pp. 172–3.
41 DPV, 4, p. 20; Hobson and Harvey, p. 31; *Letter*, p. 173.
42 DPV, 4, p. 28; Hobson and Harvey, pp. 38–9.

> would have no hesitation in accusing me of irreligion, as though it were down to me to make the blind perceive things in a manner other than that in which they perceive them.[43]

There are layers of *præteritio* here. The refusal to disclose the nature of blind metaphysics itself discloses their irreligious nature, and the instruction to the reader as to how not to read his text implicitly tells her how to. *** describes the way of reading of those who 'see crime everywhere'. It is a method informed by suspicion, not to say criminalizing paranoia, and it makes the meaning of a text depend on the reputation of its writer: the characters in the text are assumed to be mouthpieces for the writer, should the latter have a reputation for irreligion. Of course, in describing this suspicious way of reading, *** also hints to Madame that he does, in fact, have a reputation for irreligion. And this tempts us in turn to read suspiciously – a temptation that is strengthened by the phrase 'as though it were down to me', which offers her the possibility that it might indeed be down to him. In fact, *** does not so much dismiss the suspicious mode of reading as ironically authorize it, but on one condition, namely that if he were to provide the details of blind metaphysics and if Madame were to take the author to be ventriloquizing his own views through blind men, she be not scandalized but amused. Here, then, not only does *** ironically authorize us to take blind men's views on metaphysics, should he ever report any, to be his own, but he also identifies himself for the first time in the *Letter* as a writer with a reputation for irreligion. In short, he is letting us know that we should keep our eyes peeled for amusing and irreligious crime because it might indeed be everywhere.

That little game of verbal hide-and-seek lays the ground for *** to observe what he describes as an entirely uncontentious view, 'une chose dont, je crois qu'il faut que tout le monde convienne' [one observation with which I believe everyone must agree].[44] Our eyes are peeled; it is as follows: 'ce grand raisonnement, qu'on tire des merveilles de la nature, est bien faible pour des aveugles' [the grand argument that is derived from nature's marvels is very weak for the blind].[45] The claim that natural theology does not convince the blind was lurking, as we saw, in La Mothe Le Vayer's 'little treatise', in which Dreux La Vallée was reported to say that he has no idea of nature's marvels. Here in the *Letter*, it is the first explicit sign that blind men might tend towards atheism: if the truth of Christianity is considered to be demonstrable on the basis of the empirical evidence of the senses, the blind man will never have any more access to the idea of God than he will to the idea of colour. ***'s develops the

43 *Letter*, p. 180.
44 DPV, 4, p. 28; Hobson and Harvey, p. 39; *Letter*, p. 180.
45 DPV, 4, p. 28; Hobson and Harvey, p. 39; *Letter*, p. 180.

blind view, which is perhaps also his own, in a manner that is deliberately ambiguous and contains a striking paradox:

> La facilité que nous avons de créer, pour ainsi dire, de nouveaux objets, par le moyen d'une petite glace, est quelque chose de plus incompréhensible pour eux, que des astres qu'ils ont été condamnés à ne voir jamais. Ce globe lumineux qui s'avance d'orient en occident, les étonne moins qu'un petit feu qu'ils ont la commodité d'augmenter ou de diminuer: comme ils voient la matière d'une manière beaucoup plus abstraite que nous, ils sont moins éloignés de croire qu'elle pense.[46]

> The ease with which we create, as it were, new objects by means of a little mirror is something more incomprehensible to them than the stars, which they have been condemned never to see. That luminous globe that moves from east to west is less astonishing to them than a little fire which they can increase or decrease at their own convenience, for since they see matter in a much more abstract way than we do, they are less unlikely to believe it can think.[47]

This series of claims about the blind in general requires some close analysis. Certainly it is no straightforward endorsement of what seems to be their atheist and materialist metaphysics.

The numerous remarks relating to wonder and amazement in the text come into focus here, and the blind point of view is apparently belittled. What the blind find astounding is not creation with its stars and sun, but the sighted ability to 'create' objects by means of 'little' mirrors. This momentarily suggests that the blind might view the sighted as creators or gods, but the blind are also less astonished by the solar orbit and the resulting differences in temperature between night and day than they are by their own ability to increase the heat of the 'little fire' in the hearth (presumably using a pair of bellows). The blind focus resolutely on the sphere of human activities – the world, as it were, at hand – and if what astonishes them appears wholly unastonishing to the sighted, the suggestion – visible to our newly suspicious gaze – is that what seems marvellous to the sighted might not be so from another point of view.

***'s claim that the blind have been 'condemned never to see' (rather than simply 'cannot see') the marvels of creation is striking. It both recalls and subtly revises the earlier anecdote about the man-born-blind of Puiseaux being immune to punishment. Whereas he took some pleasure

46 DPV, 4, p. 28; Hobson and Harvey, p. 39.
47 *Letter*, p. 180.

in pointing out to the magistrate who wished to condemn him to imprisonment for the assault on his brother that he had been living in a dungeon all his life, and that he had no desire to be able to see, here *** expresses the view that congenital blindness is akin to congenital condemnation: if the magistrate couldn't punish him, it was because he was a man-born-punished, and if the sun and the stars suggest to the sighted the existence of a divine Creator, the fact that the blind cannot see them suggests that the Creator is a judge who has condemned the blind. Nothing is said here about the nature of divine justice, however, and any discussion of the blindness of that justice or of human blindness to its laws is postponed until later.

In the final clause, *** reports a further dimension to blind men's astonishment at the effect of their bellows: if they are amazed at their ability to control the fire, it is because, as a warm body, the fire seems to them to be alive and therefore capable of thought. So the blind are not only unimpressed by the argument from design, but they are also unlikely to believe in the existence of an immaterial soul since, in their view, matter might be able to move and think for itself. From their perspective, using bellows on a fire is not just the haptic equivalent of using a lens to make an object appear larger; it seems to them to have a real effect on a living being's body – presumably they are surprised it does not cry out. Their view is once again presented by *** as dependent on their lack of sight, but what has come to be known as the 'thinking-matter hypothesis' could also be found elsewhere in the period in texts in the sceptical and atheist tradition.

The hypothesis emerged in England in the late seventeenth century.[48] It was perhaps most strongly associated with Locke, who claimed in the *Essay Concerning Human Understanding* that while we may have an idea of thought and an idea of matter, we cannot know whether God has 'given to some Systems of Matter, fitly disposed, a power to perceive and think, or else joined and fixed to Matter, so disposed, a thinking immaterial Substance.'[49] For Locke, it is an example of the limits of human understanding – we cannot know whether matter can think or not. However, once the *Essay* became available in France, the thinking-matter hypothesis swiftly acquired much stronger atheist connotations in clandestine manuscripts such as the *Dissertation sur la formation du monde* [Dissertation on the Formation of the World] (c. 1738) and the early version of the letter on Locke in Voltaire's *Lettres philosophiques*, and in print too, most notably in La Mettrie's *Histoire naturelle de l'âme* [Natural

48 See John W. Yolton, *Thinking Matter: Materialism in Eighteenth-Century Britain* (Oxford: Basil Blackwell, 1984); Thomson, *Bodies of Thought*.

49 Locke, *Essay*, pp. 540–1.

History of the Soul] (1745) and *L'Homme machine* [Machine Man].[50]

Its formulation in the *Letter* is most peculiar, however: *** says it depends on a 'more abstract' view of matter.[51] Why that should be the case, and quite what 'more abstract' might mean are questions that go unanswered at this stage in the *Letter* – we will explore them in the next chapter. As it is presented here, the claim has all the air of a paradox: most philosophers claimed precisely the opposite – that is, they argued that a tendency to think in abstractions either proceeded from a dualist premise, that is, a belief in a body and a soul, or produced dualist results: non-thinking matter and thinking non-matter. Because of this, supporters of the thinking matter hypothesis tended to be highly critical of abstract thought. Hobbes, for instance, had complained in *De Corpore* [On the Body] (1655) that:

> [S]ome men seeing they can consider [. . .] accidents, without considering their bodies or subjects (which they call *abstracting,* or making to exist apart by themselves), they speak of accidents, as if they might be separated from all bodies. And from hence proceed the gross errors of writers of metaphysics; for, because they can consider thought without the consideration of body, they infer there is no need of a thinking-body.[52]

And La Mettrie made a similar point in the *Histoire naturelle de l'âme* [Natural History of the Soul] (1745): 'quelques philosophes ont pensé que l'âme n'est ni matière, ni corps, parce que considérant la matière par abstraction, ils l'envisagaient douée seulement de propriétés passives et mécaniques' [some philosophers have thought that the soul is neither matter nor body because, thinking of matter in abstract terms, they envisaged it as possessing only passive and mechanical properties].[53] *** seems, therefore, to have the blind come close to a conclusion, namely that matter can think, which their more abstract way of thinking ought to preclude. If the sighted are astonished at creation, the reader is astonished at ***'s claim.

A further layer of peculiarity is perhaps to be found in the fact that it

---

50 Timo Kaitaro, *Diderot's Holism* (Frankfurt am Main: Peter Lang, 1997), pp. 86–90.

51 Bourdin has also observed that it is 'remarquable' [remarkable] (*Diderot. Le matérialisme*, p. 40), but he tends to want to explain away its strangeness (pp. 39–43).

52 Thomas Hobbes, *The English Works of Thomas Hobbes, now first collected and edited by Sir William Molesworth*, 11 volumes (London: J. Bohn, 1839–45), vol. 1, pp. 33–4.

53 Julien Offray de La Mettrie, *Histoire naturelle de l'âme traduite de l'anglois de M. Charp, par M. H** de l'Académie des sciences. Nouvelle édition revue fort exactement, corrigée de quantité de fautes & augmentée de la lettre critique de M. de la Mettrie à Madame la marquise du Châtelet* (Oxford [Paris]: Aux dépends de l'auteur, 1747), p. 280.

was not only materialist thinkers who were critical of abstract thought for producing dualist results. Berkeley, a thinker in whose work the Encyclopedists took much interest, deeming it to be the height of sceptical paradoxes,[54] reversed Hobbes' view and argued that metaphysicians had been erroneously led to infer the existence of body because they had considered it in the abstract, separately from the mind that perceives it. In *A Treatise Concerning the Principles of Human Knowledge* (1710), Berkeley claimed that the belief in the separate existence of material substance will 'be found to depend on the doctrine of abstract ideas'.[55] Certainly he does not explicitly argue that, in addition to a belief in the existence of matter, abstract thought results in a belief that it can think, for his aim is to dispense with matter completely so as to short-circuit any discussion of what its capabilities might be. Yet *** will later make reference to Berkeley's *Three Dialogues between Hylas and Philonous* (1713),[56] which had been translated by the Encyclopedist, Gua de Malves,[57] and so although Berkeley's name is absent here, it might not be impossible to see the conclusion at which the blind arrive as one that Berkeleyan metaphysics predicts – abstraction leads to materialism – but which it attempts to eradicate.

Our eyes are peeled for further references, paradoxical or otherwise, to thinking matter and abstract thought. They come later. Now, and rather suddenly, the text operates a volte-face as *** shifts register and treats Madame to a spectacular play on the connotations of blindness and sight.

See and Tell

What *** says is worth quoting at length in order to grasp the changing connotations, literal and metaphorical, positive and negative, of sight and blindness:

> Si un homme qui n'a vu que pendant un jour ou deux, se trouvait confondu chez un peuple d'aveugles, il faudrait qu'il prît le parti de se taire, ou celui de passer pour un fou. Il leur annoncerait tous les jours quelque nouveau mystère qui n'en serait un que pour eux,

54 See H. M. Bracken, *The Early Reception of Berkeley's Immaterialism, 1710–1733* (The Hague: Nijhoff, 1959); Sébastien Charles, *Berkeley au siècle des Lumières: immatérialisme et scepticisme au XVIIIe siècle*, preface by Geneviève Brykman (Paris: Vrin, 2003).

55 George Berkeley, *A Treatise Concerning the Principles of Human Knowledge*, Jonathan Dancy (ed.) (Oxford: Oxford University Press, 1998), p. 104.

56 In the *Dialogues*, published three years after the *Principles*, the character Philonous puts forward the same argument as that of the *Principles*.

57 It had for a long time been claimed that the text was first translated in 1750, but Sébastien Charles has recently identified an earlier one, dating from 1744 (see 'De Popkin à Rousseau: retour sur le scepticisme des Lumières'. *Philosophiques*, 35.1 (2008), 275–90, p. 284, note 34).

> et que les esprits forts se sauraient bon gré de ne pas croire. Les défenseurs de la religion ne pourraient-ils pas tirer un grand parti d'une incrédulité si opiniâtre, si juste même à certains égards, et cependant si peu fondée?[58]
>
> If a man who had only been able to see for a day or two were to find himself lost in a land of the blind, he would have to decide between keeping quiet and being taken for a madman. Every day, he would proclaim some new mystery, which would only be a mystery to the blind and which the freethinkers would pride themselves on not believing. Could the defenders of religion not make good use of such stubborn and, to some extent, such fair, and yet such ill-founded unbelief?[59]

Here we have a hypothetical variation on the cataract narrative in which to acquire sight is no longer to accede to the same experiences as other people, but to gain an extra sense. Initially, the fact that the man has 'only' been able to see for a day or two suggests the saying 'In the kingdom of the blind, the one-eyed man is king', but this man risks ostracism rather than glory in announcing what he can see. As such, this hypothetical man, who was once blind but is now able to see, sounds like a figure for Christ or Paul, an echo that is confirmed by the subsequent reference to the defenders of religion. Following the report of blind metaphysics, the text seems to have lurched into some highly orthodox symbolism, retrospectively confirming that blind metaphysics posed a serious challenge.

That the passage can be read in orthodox ways is confirmed by its quotability. 0 concludes his *Encyclopédie* article 'Blind Man' with these lines, introducing them with the phrase '[n]ous terminerons cet article par cette réflexion, capable d'en contrebalancer quelques autres qui se trouvent répandues dans l'ouvrage, et qui ne sont pas tout à fait si orthodoxes' [we shall conclude this article with this observation which is able to counterbalance some others which are spread throughout the work and which are not quite so orthodox]. And some years later, the Catholic apologist, Bergier, would also quote it in the service of Catholic doctrine, arguing in *Le Déisme réfuté par lui-même* [Deism Refuted on its Own Terms] (1765) that just as the blind have no choice but to believe the sighted when they speak of colours, so they must also believe the sighted when they speak

---

58 DPV, 4, p. 28; Hobson and Harvey, p. 39.

59 *Letter*, p. 180.

of the marvels of nature.[60] Bergier omits, however, the final reference to the 'defenders of religion' and he is surely right to do so: located in an interrogative in which 'unbelief' is rather equivocally condemned – 'such stubborn and, to some extent, such fair, and yet such ill-founded unbelief' – the apology he might build on the basis of the Christ-figure's words and the blind reaction to them is at best rather wobbly. The *Encyclopédie* article, by contrast, deliberately ends on it.

The paragraph wobbles again as the first 'if' clause is swiftly followed by another that undermines its (relative) orthodoxy. *** goes on:

> Si vous vous prêtez pour un instant à cette supposition, elle vous rappellera sous des traits empruntés l'histoire et les persécutions de ceux qui ont eu le malheur de rencontrer la vérité dans des siècles de ténèbres, et l'imprudence de la déceler à leurs aveugles contemporains, entre lesquels ils n'ont point eu d'ennemis plus cruels que ceux qui par leur état et leur éducation semblaient devoir être les moins éloignés de leurs sentiments.[61]

> If you entertain that supposition for a moment, it will bring to mind in another guise the history and persecutions of those who were unlucky enough to discover the truth in the dark ages and unwise enough to reveal it to their blind contemporaries, among whom they had no crueller enemies than those whose order and education ought, it seemed, to have made them hold the least dissimilar views.[62]

The first hypothesis, presented by d'Alembert as counterbalancing others to be found elsewhere in the *Letter*, is also thus counterbalanced by another. This one invites us to read the first hypothetical story of the man who saw the light and whose revelations were accepted as mysterious by the blind, but rejected by the dogmatic freethinkers, as an allegory for real men in history – Galileo, perhaps Vanini – who saw the light and were not so much disbelieved by dogmatic freethinkers who thought they were mad as cruelly persecuted by an educated but dogmatic and non-freethinking clergy. Bergier's refutation steers well clear of this, of course, as does the *Encyclopédie* article, but any reader of those texts familiar enough with the *Letter* to know how it goes on could not fail to

---

60 Hisayasu Nakagawa, 'Diderot, Rousseau et autres "incrédules" au service du catholicisme: à propos du *Déisme réfuté par lui-même* de l'abbé Bergier'. *Recherches sur Diderot et l'Encyclopédie*, 39 (2005), 157–76, 162–3.

61 DPV, 4, p. 28; Hobson and Harvey, p. 39.

62 *Letter*, p. 180.

recognize (and be amused by) what we can now clearly see are the text's deliberately contrarian dynamics.

If it is clear, then, that the blind tend to hold atheist views, and if it is suggested that *** might share them, what exactly is involved in their 'more abstract' way of thinking remains unexplained. It will be clarified in the next section of the *Letter*, in which *** seems to share not only the views of the blind, but also their way of thinking as he closes his eyes and begins to talk to Madame about his sense of touch.

Four

Groping Around in the Light

That the *Letter* is entering a new phase is clearly signalled by *** when he announces, 'Je laisse donc la morale et la métaphysique des aveugles, et je passe à des choses qui sont moins importantes, mais qui tiennent de plus près au but des observations qu'on fait ici de toutes parts, depuis l'arrivée du Prussien' [So I leave behind the morality and metaphysics of the blind and move on to less important things, but ones that are more closely related to the point of all the observations people are constantly making these days ever since the Prussian arrived].[1] He is turning to Molyneux's Problem or, rather, to 'Question one', which involves, we recall, whether a man-born-blind could gain the ideas of a cube and a sphere through his touch. This change of focus is accompanied by a shift in the status of the man-born-blind: ***'s conception of the manner in which the blind acquire their ideas – his sense of whether they have imaginations and what their memories are like – is not so much based on the evidence of a real man-born-blind as on his own experience. *** explores his perceptions and ideas as a sighted man, but also as one who can be blind, that is, who can close his eyes and rely on his sense of touch.

This part of the *Letter*, which comes after the narrative recounting the visit to Puiseaux and ***'s speculations regarding blind metaphysics but before the supposed translation of Inchlif's account of Saunderson's deathbed conversation with his vicar, has received little critical attention.[2] This is not only because it also involves some quite lengthy arithmetical calculations but it is also because the argument makes some disconcerting moves. The Index to the *Letter* retrospectively confirms the surprising and contradictory shape of the argument: the entry 'Aveugles-nés' [Blind, men, born] has two contradictory sub-entries, 'sont enclins au matérialisme' [are inclined to materialism] and 'sont enclins à l'idéalisme' [are inclined to idealism].[3] The first sends the reader to the end of the section

1 DPV, 4, p. 28; Hobson and Harvey, p. 39; *Letter*, pp. 180–1.
2 Colas Duflo is an exception once again, though his approach and his conclusions are quite different to mine (see *Diderot philosophe*, pp. 91–4, 135–9).
3 DPV, 4, p. 73; Hobson and Harvey, p. 83; *Letter*, p. 220.

studied in the previous chapter, where *** does indeed report the tendency of the blind to materialist beliefs; the second sends the reader to the end of the section that will be studied here and which concludes, as we'll see, with the claim that the blind tend to accept the Berkeleyan denial of the existence of material substance.

Another important aspect to this section of the *Letter* is the series of remarks about blind men's use of language, which puts forward a theory of verbal allusion. It receives my attention here and it informs the close reading that follows inasmuch as I try to unearth the possible allusions contained in a turn of phrase that *** himself rather allusively describes as 'ingenious'. Before doing so, however, I turn to the peculiarities of ***'s attempt to present his own experience, be it visual or haptic, as epistemologically exemplary, and to the shifting relationships between blindness and touch as they relate to abstract thought.

Imagination and Memory

*** claims that a blind man could gain ideas of straight and curved lines through his sense of touch, by passing a taut or loose piece of string through his fingers. He observes in passing that the blind man need not be a geometer – an intriguing detail, the importance of which will not emerge until much later – and explores instead the differences between an idea gained in this haptic way and one acquired through sight. To obtain an idea through touch, the subject is required, *** says, to remember a sequence of impressions. This is not the case in visual perception, which operates in an instant. He concludes, then, that the mental faculty on which a blind man would seem to rely is his memory.[4] The sighted, by contrast, rely on their imaginations – a faculty that a blind man either lacks or of which he can make no use, since he has no ideas of colour and light. *** boldly asserts:

> il ne se passe rien dans sa tête d'analogue à ce qui se passe dans la nôtre; il n'imagine point, car pour imaginer il faut colorer un fond, et détacher de ce fond des points, en leur supposant une couleur différente de celle du fond. Restituez à ces points la même couleur qu'au fond; à l'instant ils se confondent avec lui, et la figure disparaît; du moins, c'est ainsi que les choses s'exécutent dans mon imagination, et je présume que les autres n'imaginent pas autrement que moi.[5]

> nothing happens in his head the way it does in ours because he cannot imagine, since to imagine, you must colour in a background

4 DPV, 4, p. 29; Hobson and Harvey, p. 40; *Letter*, p. 181.
5 DPV, 4, p. 29; Hobson and Harvey, p. 40.

> and make some points stand out against it by supposing them to be of a different colour. If you make the points the same colour as the background, they immediately merge together and the shape disappears; at least, that's how things happen in my imagination and I presume other people don't imagine any differently.[6]

***'s logic has a peculiar relationship to the process of inductive reasoning, which he earlier said was faulty: while he starts by recognising that what goes on inside us is not the same as what goes on inside the blind man, he then overrides the possibility of any difference between sighted people and presents his own imagination as exemplary. Yet his description of what it is like to imagine is very strikingly painterly, and while this emphasises the radical difference between the sighted mind and the blind mind, his claim that *all* sighted readers imagine in this painterly way is questionable. Indeed the text itself calls it into question – ***'s caveat, 'at least that's what happens in my imagination', suggests he is aware that his imagination might not a representative example. His attempt to set himself up as the exemplary sighted person who is able to speak for all readers is not without irony; in fact, it rather has the effect of placing the sighted reader in his shadow.

If few sighted people imagine in the kind of technicolour that *** does, they do nonetheless think in their imaginations. The blind, by contrast, so *** claims, think in their memories, working with haptic impressions that the sighted tend simply to forget:

> Si cette mémoire est très fugitive en nous, si nous n'avons guère d'idée de la manière dont un aveugle-né fixe, rappelle et combine les sensations du toucher, c'est une suite de l'habitude que nous avons prise par les yeux, de tout exécuter dans notre imagination avec des couleurs. Il m'est cependant arrivé à moi-même, dans les agitations d'une passion violente, d'éprouver un frissonnement dans toute une main; de sentir l'impression de corps que j'avais touchés il y avait longtemps, s'y réveiller aussi vivement que s'ils eussent encore été présents à mon attouchement, et de m'apercevoir très distinctement que les limites de la sensation coïncidaient précisément avec celles de ces corps absents.[7]

> If this memory is very fleeting in us and we barely have any idea how a blind man grasps, remembers and combines the sensations of touch, it is because our eyes have put us in the habit of doing

6 *Letter*, p. 181.
7 DPV, 4, p. 30; Hobson and Harvey, p. 41.

> everything with colours in our imaginations. I have myself, however, had the experience of being in the grip of a violent passion and felt my whole hand tremble as the impressions of bodies that I had touched a long time ago were reawakened in me as vividly as if they were still present to my touch, and I could very clearly perceive an exact correlation between the outlines of my sensation and those of these absent bodies.[8]

Once again, *** is an exception to the sighted rule: he may not be blind but he has very strong memories of haptic impressions; they seem to be as vivid as the visual images in his imagination. *** is, as it were, in touch with the blind.

Furthermore, his tingling fingers suggest to him that it is only because we are born sighted that we think in our heads; perhaps a man-born-blind would think somewhere else. To test this hypothesis, he comes up with a thought experiment involving a man-born-blind-and-deaf, a man, that is, with no sensory organs of any epistemological significance in his head.[9] He speculates as follows:

> Si jamais un philosophe aveugle et sourd de naissance fait un homme à l'imitation de celui de Descartes, j'ose vous assurer, Madame, qu'il placera l'âme au bout des doigts; car c'est de là que lui viennent ses principales sensations, et toutes ses connaissances. Et qui l'avertirait que sa tête est le siège de ses pensées? Si les travaux de l'imagination épuisent la nôtre, c'est que l'effort que nous faisons pour imaginer, est assez semblable à celui que nous faisons pour apercevoir des objets très proches ou très petits. Mais il n'en sera pas de même de l'aveugle et sourd de naissance; [. . .] je ne serais pas surpris qu'après une profonde méditation, il eût les doigts aussi fatigués, que nous avons la tête.[10]

> If a philosopher who was born blind and deaf were ever to come up with a man on Descartes' model, I dare say, Madame, he would place the soul in the fingertips because they are the source of his principal sensations and all of his knowledge. And who would tell him that his head is the main seat of his thoughts? If our heads find the labours of the imagination exhausting, it's because the effort of

8 *Letter*, p. 182.

9 Smell and taste are not usually accorded any great role in empiricist epistemologies. Diderot's *Pensées sur l'interprétation de la nature* [Thoughts on the Interpretation of Nature] (1753) will describe scientific speculations in terms of smell. See DPV, 9, p. 48.

10 DPV, 4, pp. 31–2; Hobson and Harvey, p. 42.

> imagining is quite similar to that of perceiving objects that are very close to us or very small. But it's not like that for the man-born-blind-and-deaf. [. . .] I wouldn't be surprised if thinking deeply left his fingertips as tired as it does our heads.[11]

Such a man would not, he says, locate his mind, as Descartes had done, in the pineal gland – a kind of third, inner eye; he would instead locate it in the ends of his fingers, because they are the primary organs of touch.[12] The location of the mind thus appears relative, dependent on which sensory organ is dominant in the body The claim can also be found in *Les Bijoux Indiscrets*, in which Mangogul, the sex-obsessed sultan, is said to believe that women's minds are located in their vaginas.[13]

Yet whether the mind is in the head or the hands or anywhere else in the body, the assumption seems to be that the mind is physical and that thinking is a property of matter. What then of the earlier claim that the view of matter as capable of thought depended on a 'more abstract' way of thinking?

Touch and Drawing

It is perhaps not immediately obvious that the man-born-blind-and-deaf's sore fingers are doing more abstract work than the sighted man's sore head, nor do ***'s convulsive frissons immediately seem more abstract than his mental paintings. However, the relationship between blindness and abstraction is now restated. *** claims that since the blind do not think in images, they think in more abstract ways:

> Mais si l'imagination d'un aveugle n'est autre chose que la faculté de se rappeler et de combiner des sensations de points palpables, et celle d'un homme qui voit, la faculté de se rappeler et de combiner des points visibles ou colorés, il s'ensuit que l'aveugle-né aperçoit les choses d'une manière beaucoup plus abstraite que nous [. . .] Car l'abstraction ne consiste qu'à séparer par la pensée les qualités

11 *Letter*, p. 183.

12 *** also refers to the blind mind as 'le sens interne' [the inner sense]. If *** uses this Aristotelian term here, it is not to suggest that there is a 'sensorium commune', in which the different sensory impressions come together. Colas Duflo has rightly refuted this claim (*Diderot philosophe*, p. 96) made by Yvon Belaval (DPV, 4, p. 81, note 34). *** does so instead because of the strong haptic connotations of the 'inner sense' (see Heller-Roazen, *The Inner Touch*, pp. 31–42). The inner sense was also of interest to a number of late seventeenth- and early eighteenth-century English and French materialists – La Mettrie, for example, identified it with the physical organ of the brain (see Thomson, *Bodies of Thought*, pp. 199–201).

13 DPV, 3, p. 98.

> sensibles des corps, ou les unes des autres, ou du corps même qui leur sert de base[.][14]

> Yet if a blind man's imagination is nothing other than the faculty of recalling and combining the sensations of palpable points and that of a man who can see, the faculty of recalling and combining visible or coloured points, it follows that the man who is blind from birth perceives things in a much more abstract manner than we do. [. . .] since abstraction consists simply in mentally separating the sensible qualities of bodies either from each other or from the body that underlies them[.][15]

The point seems to be that whereas the visible points, with which the sighted think, involve qualities that come from more than one sense (sight as well as touch), the palpable points, with which the blind think, are made up of ideas that come from one sense alone.[16] Visual perception is thus complex and haptic perception simple, and on these grounds, the blind think in more abstract ways than the sighted – not, we note, in an entirely abstract way.[17] If touch thus seems to be understood as the simplest form of sensory perception, on which visual perception builds, adding light and colour, this would indicate two important intertexts: the *Cours de Peinture par principes* [The Principles of Painting] (1709), by the painter and theorist, Roger de Piles, and Berkeley's *New Theory of Vision* (1709).

If *** describes the sighted imagination as painting, he also suggests that the haptic memory is akin to drawing.[18] A comparison between blind men and draughtsmen may sound paradoxical inasmuch as drawing is a form of visual representation, but it can be found in contemporaneous art

---

14 DPV, 4, p. 32; Hobson and Harvey, p. 42.

15 *Letter*, p. 183.

16 I am following Bourdin here (*Diderot. Le matérialisme*, p. 41).

17 I depart from Bourdin's view here; he states: 'L'aveugle abstrait, non par volonté, mais spontanément, par un effet nécessaire de la reduction de son imagination à la seule combinaison de sensations tactiles, au lieu que la vue nous donne à percevoir des objets dont les qualités, provenant en outre de différents sens qui se prêtent mutuellement secours, sont difficilement séparables les unes des autres' [The blind man abstracts not by will but spontaneously and as a necessary effect of the fact that his imagination is necessarily reduced to combining tactile sensations, whereas sight allows us to perceive objects whose qualities are harder to separate from each other, not least because they come from the different senses, working together]. (*Diderot. Le matérialisme*, p. 41).

18 See also Derrida, *Memoirs of the Blind*.

theory, which we also know Diderot to have been reading.[19] As Jacqueline Lichtenstein has shown, the comparison first appeared in Piles' *Cours de Peinture par principes*, a work of anti-Cartesian art theory, arguing for the superiority of colour over line.[20] Cartesian theorists, such as Le Brun, had elevated line over colour on the grounds that the former was abstract, ideal and geometrical, while the latter was material and appealed to the physical senses. Piles argued, in opposition, that both line and colour appealed to the senses, and that since sight was the noblest of the senses and touch the lowest, colour was superior, because even the ignoble blind were capable of sensing line by running their hands over a sculpture. Colour, however, escaped blind men's grasp.[21] Some of these ideas also echo in the *Letter*, in which *** accepts the Pilesian association of touch with line: we recall how *** spoke of how he could feel a 'correlation between the *outlines* of my sensation and those of these absent bodies' (my emphasis). *** will later refer to the pleasures the blind could take in sculpture,[22] and imagine a draughtsman drawing a portrait on the palm of Madame's hand while she has her eyes closed.[23] However, Piles's view that touch is inferior to sight and line to colour is much less obviously present; indeed, if the *Letter* accepts the anti-Cartesian association between touch and line, it is for purposes that neither Piles nor Descartes would endorse: it seeks positively to suggest that the intellect is material by associating it with touch.[24]

Berkeley did not, of course, accept that the mind was material any more than Descartes did; indeed, he went far beyond Descartes to argue that the very existence of material substance was an illusion. However, his conception of the sense of touch is nonetheless important for the *Letter*, precisely because of its anti-Cartesianism. It is to be found in *A New Theory of Vision*, which made an important contribution to Molyneux's Problem and which Diderot knew, if not directly, then through Voltaire's *Eléments de la*

19 He borrowed the *Cours de peinture* from the Bibliothèque du roi in January 1748 (Proust, 'L'Initiation artistique de Diderot', p. 230).

20 See Jacqueline Lichtenstein, *La Couleur éloquente: rhétorique et peinture à l'âge classique* (Paris: Flammarion, 1989), pp. 153–82; *The Eloquence of Colour: Rhetoric and Painting in the French Classical Age*, Emily McVarish (trans.) (Berkeley: University of California Press, 1993), pp. 138–68. See also Bernard Teyssèdre, *Roger de Piles et les débats sur le coloris au siècle de Louis XIV* (Paris: Bibliothèque des Arts, 1964).

21 Roger de Piles, *Cours de peinture par principes* (Paris: Jombert, 1766), pp. 259–63.

22 DPV, 4, p. 46; Hobson and Harvey, pp. 57–8; *Letter*, pp. 197–8.

23 DPV, 4, pp. 47–48; Hobson and Harvey, pp. 58–9; *Letter*, p. 198

24 For Lichtenstein, the *Letter* is Cartesian in its allegiances. See *La Tache aveugle: essai sur les relations de la peinture et de la sculpture à l'âge moderne* (Paris: Gallimard, 2003), pp. 92–3; *The Blind Spot: An Essay on the Relations Between Painting and Sculpture in the Modern Age*, Chris Miller (trans.) (Los Angeles: Getty Publications, 2008), pp. 68–9.

philosophie de Newton [Elements of Newton's Philosophy] (1738), to which the *Letter* explicitly refers.[25] The *New Theory* argues that it is not sight, as Locke had claimed, but touch that is the source of our ideas of shape, size, distance and motion. Crucially, these were the ideas that, for Descartes, were only available from the senses inasmuch as they were underpinned by geometrical abstractions that were innately present to reason.[26]

At this stage in the *Letter*, *** would seem to share Berkeley's view of the primacy of touch. He suggests, as we've seen, that our visual perception of shape involves combining ideas obtained from sight and touch, which is to say that visual perception is dependent on prior haptic perception. *** will later contradict this view of touch as the primary sense, but for the moment, he turns to consider whether there can be any ideas more abstract than those acquired haptically.

An English Geometer's Ingenious Expression

*** speaks of 'une espèce d'abstraction dont si peu d'hommes sont capables, qu'elle semble réservée aux intelligences pures' [one kind of abstraction of which so few men are capable that it seems to be reserved for pure intellects].[27] He does not yet tell us who such exceptional men might be, if they exist at all, and concentrates instead on explaining what this kind of abstraction would involve. It would reduce everything to mathematical points, and he comments:

> si, par hasard, c'était là le fondement de la doctrine de Pythagore, on pourrait dire de lui, qu'il échoua dans son projet, parce que cette manière de philosopher est trop au-dessus de nous, et trop approchante de celle de l'Être Suprême qui, selon l'expression ingénieuse d'un géomètre anglais, *géométrise* perpétuellement dans l'univers.[28]

> if, by chance, this was the basis for Pythagoras's doctrine, we could say of him that he failed in his project because that kind of philosophizing is too far beyond us and much closer to that of the Supreme Being who, according to the ingenious expression of an English geometer, is perpetually *geometrizing* in the universe.[29]

What are we to make of this reference to the 'Supreme Being'? Certainly, the English geometer's expression is striking, and *** clearly wishes to

25 DPV, 4, p. 60; Hobson and Harvey, p. 70; *Letter*, p. 209.
26 Berkeley, *A New Theory of Vision*, pp. 49–50.
27 DPV, 4, p. 33; Hobson and Harvey, p. 43. *Letter*, p. 184.
28 DPV, 4, p. 33; Hobson and Harvey, p. 43.
29 *Letter*, p. 184.

ensure we find it so by describing it as 'ingenious', italicizing the verb and elliptically referring to 'an English geometer' whose identity is withheld, though the reference to his nationality ensures that we do not think it is Descartes. Moreover, the phrase follows on from a passing reference to Pythagoras who, in addition to his numerical theories, was known for his 'esoteric' expressions that were designed to veil their meaning from the uninitiated.[30] Something is clearly afoot: is it a further opportunity to read through eyes that see crime everywhere?

The Geometer-God is a topos of Neo-Pythagorean and Neo-Platonic thought, and it can be found in a number of early modern discussions of mathematics. In Bayle's dictionary, for example, the article 'Zénon l'Epicurien' [Zeno the Epicurean] quotes the phrase 'Deum semper geometriam tractare' [God is always performing geometry] from Plutarch's *Life of Marcellus* in the course of a discussion of the Neo-Platonic view of mathematics, according to which it takes us away from the material world of sensible objects in which we are blind, and into the luminous world of pure ideas.[31] As a philosophical commonplace, it is hardly 'ingenious'. However, in an English context, the Geometer-God easily acquires 'criminal' associations.

The English Geometer-God is to be understood as that of deism, of rational religion, in which God's movements can be described according to the laws of mathematics. He is not the Biblical God of mercy nor is he the author of miracles, which were understood by the deists to be impossible, merely signs of the observer's limited understanding. Indeed, inasmuch as the Supreme Being is thought to be both perpetually maintaining order and symmetry in the universe and sublimely impervious to human suffering, he is ironically prefigured by the man-born-blind of Puiseaux who, we recall, was forever tidying his house in the dark and could only perceive the suffering of others if it was audible, and even then was liable not to respond. But why the cryptic reference to the 'English geometer'?

The writings of one particularly notable English geometer, Newton, are marked by the Neo-Platonic belief that the study of mathematics can give us access to the eternal truths that exist in God's mind.[32] However, the specific italicized phrase does not appear in Newton and, as in many a

---

30 See 'Pythagorisme' [Pythagorisme] in *Encyclopédie*, vol. 13, pp. 614–31.

31 Pierre Bayle, *Dictionnaire historique et critique*, fifth edition, 4 volumes (Amsterdam, Leiden, The Hague, Utrecht, 1740), vol. 4, p. 548.

32 Saunderson's *Elements* ends with a similar pæan to his discipline (*Elements*, vol. 2, pp. 740–2). A good survey of the question of Newton's beliefs can be found in Scott Mandelbrote, 'Newton and Eighteenth-Century Christianity' in *The Cambridge Companion to Newton*, I. Bernard Cohen and George E. Smith (eds) (Cambridge: Cambridge University Press, 2002), pp. 409–30.

modern quizbook, the answer is given at the back: as observed earlier, the *Letter* has an Index, compiled by Diderot, and it reveals that the English geometer in question is 'Rapson' or, more accurately, Joseph Raphson, the Cambridge mathematician. His *De Spatio reali* [Of Real Space] (1697), an appendix to his Newtonian work on infinite series, ends with the lines:

> Minimam quidem muscam, vel vegetabilium simplicissimam, theoreticè componere humana Philosophia nescit, aæquè ac practicè potentia nequit; multò minus totum componere Universum. Problemata sunt, primordiali Sapientiâ, & Potentiâ, rerum productrice, digna, et Cognitionis ulteriorem progressionem in æternum usq. nobis suppeditent, tam ipsarum rerum, quàm perpetuò geometrizantis in universo DEI.[33]

> Human philosophy can neither theoretically compose the smallest mouse nor the simplest plant, nor can human praxis build them, much less the whole universe. These are problems worthy of the Primordial Wisdom and Power, which produces these things. As for us, they offer us only a progress in æternum of our knowledge both of the things themselves and of the perpetually geometrizing GOD.

Hobson and Harvey have rightly observed that although it is not impossible that Diderot only knew the last lines of the work, he is likely to have known that *De Spatio reali* was suspected of atheism, largely owing to its claim that God shared the same qualities as space.[34] In his *Letters to Serena* (1704), Toland, the radical freethinker, said of Raphson and others,[35] on whose work he drew:

---

33 Joseph Raphson, *Analysis æquationum universalis, seu, Ad æquationes algebraicas resolvendas methodus generalis, & expedita, ex nova infinitarum serierum methodo, deducta ac demonstrata. Editio secunda cum appendice; cui annexum est, De spatio reali, seu entre infinito conamen mathematico-metaphysicum* (London: Typis T. Braddyll, prostant venales apud Johannem Taylor, 1697), p. 95. For studies of Raphson, see Alexander Koyré, *From the Closed World to the Infinite Universe* (New York: Harper, 1958), pp. 140–50; Brian T. Copenhaver, 'Jewish Theologies of Space in the Scientific Revolution: Henry More, Joseph Raphson, Isaac Newton and their Predecessors'. *Annals of Science*, 37.5 (1980), 489–548.

34 Hobson and Harvey, p. 221. Berkeley takes Raphson to be a materialist along with Hobbes, Spinoza and Locke (see 'Philosophical Commentaries' in *The Works of George Berkeley, Bishop of Cloyne*, A. A. Luce and T. E. Jessop (eds), 9 volumes (London: Nelson, 1948–64), vol. 1, pp. 298, 825).

35 They include Lucretius, Bruno, Campanella, Hobbes, Descartes, More, Gassendi and Spinoza.

> I am satisfied that most of those Gentlemen did firmly believe in the existence of a deity, and I charitably hope it of 'em all; but in my opinion their unwary zeal refined him into mere nothing, or (what they would as little allow) they made nature or the universe to be the only God: but the goodness of their intention ought to secure 'em with all men of candour from the charge and consequence of atheism.[36]

And in a similarly ironic vein, Toland described Raphson himself as 'ingenious'.[37] Is this a coincidence or did Diderot know this?[38] And if so, did he intend ***'s usage of the same adjective to indicate the atheist potential of the work from which it is taken?

Such questions are left unanswered as *** now turns his attention to the human realm, in which he refers to men-born-deaf-dumb-and-blind in order to argue that there is no such thing as a purely abstract idea that is not derived from sensory experience. His claim is that men-born-deaf-dumb-and-blind are not to be thought of as thinking silently in the dark, but rather as languishing in 'un état d'imbécilité' [a feeble-minded state] because they have so few functioning sense organs and therefore so few ideas.[39] And since we, the sighted and hearing, use only visible and audible means of communication, we cannot teach them. Such a dismissive attitude to men-born-deaf-dumb-and-blind is perhaps surprising, and although it confirms the importance of hearing and speaking in the *Letter*, it is also called into question by ***'s subsequent reference to palpable forms of communication and, in particular, the palpable notation invented by another Cambridge mathematician, Nicholas Saunderson.

Staying in Touch

*** presents Saunderson's highly complex method of performing calculations palpably on a machine of his own invention. It enabled him to do them at high speed, his fingers darting across with great agility, which stands in stark contrast to ***'s very lengthy explanation of how the machine worked.[40] Much of the explanation is taken from 'Dr Saunderson's Palpable Arithmetic Decypher'd', which appeared as a second preface to Saunderson's *Elements of Algebra* and was written by John Colson, Saunderson's successor to the Lucasian Chair.[41] However, *** adds

---

36 John Toland, *Letters to Serena* (London: Printed for Bernard Lintot, 1704), pp. 219–20. For an exploration of their differences, see Thomson, *Bodies of Thought*, pp. 133–4.

37 Toland, *Letters*, p. 219.

38 *Letters to Serena* was not translated into French until 1768 but it was known in France before that (see Thomson, *Bodies of Thought*, p. 197).

39 DPV, 4, p. 33; Hobson and Harvey, p. 43; *Letter*, p. 184.

40 DPV, 4, pp. 33–41; Hobson and Harvey, pp. 43–52; *Letter*, pp. 185–92.

41 Saunderson, *Elements*, vol. 1, pp. xx–xxvi.

more examples, perhaps with the aim of emphasising further the contrast between Saunderson's digital dexterity and the laboriousness of explaining it to the sighted. The *Letter* also includes, in addition to a plate taken from Colson that has been divided into two separate figures (Figures II and III), three new plates of Diderot's invention, apparently designed to aid the sighted reader's comprehension. However, the explanation of Figure III contains an error: *** says 'left' when he must mean 'right'.[42] Of course, this could simply be a mistake (and it was quite common for plates to be printed the wrong way round), but given the fondness for reversals and mirror images in the *Letter*, it is not impossible that it is deliberate, designed to test the reader's comprehension of the explanations (and perhaps her patience, given their length and repetitiveness).[43]

The *Letter*'s focus on Saunderson's palpable arithmetic may not be without a degree of polemical intent. As we've seen in relation to Raphson, English mathematicians were viewed with some suspicion. Here, what is said about Saunderson might be read in relation to the recent controversy concerning the relationships between alegebraic symbols and the entities for which they stand. Descartes had applied algebra to geometry in *La Géométrie* [Geometry] (1637), which was published together with *La Dioptrique*, but it would be the infinitesimal calculus of Newton and Leibniz, the real existence of the infinitesimals symbolized in the algebra, that would cause serious debate. And the terms of that debate made frequent use of the metaphors of blindness and sight.

In response to his critics, Leibniz boldly described the infinitesimals as 'fictions utiles' [useful fictions],[44] explaining that their utility, which was also that of signs in general, lay in their ability to free the mind from its limitations and dependence on sensible forms. Algebraic symbols led the mind towards ideas that lay beyond its natural reach and guided it as though it were a blind man, enabling what he called 'cogitatio cæca' [blind reasoning].[45] In England, Newton's use of infinitesimals, or what

42 DPV, 4, p. 38; *Lettre*, p. 49; *Letter*, p. 189.

43 For a different reading, see Michael Kessler, 'A Puzzle Concerning Diderot's Presentation of Saunderson's "Palpable Arithmetic"'. *Diderot Studies*, 20 (1981), 159–73. There may be a visual game being played in the printer's ornaments that appear on the first page [Figure 1]; they are made up of black and white squares that resemble in a more decorative mode the dots and squares of Saunderson's invention.

44 Their reality was accepted by Bernouilli, Varignon and L'Hôpital; see Douglas M. Jesseph, 'Leibniz on the Foundations of the Calculus: The Question of the Reality of Infinitesimal Magnitudes'. *Perspectives on Science*, 6.1–2 (1998), 6–40.

45 Quoted in Enrico Pasini, 'Arcanum Artis Inveniendi: Leibniz and Analysis', in *Analysis and Synthesis in Mathematics: History and Philosophy*, Michael Otte and Marco Panza (eds) (Dordrecht: Kluwer, 1997), 35–46, p. 45.

he called 'fluxions', also came under attack, most notably by Berkeley in the *Analyst* (1734).[46] Berkeley argued that infinitesimals were inconceivable, famously describing them as 'Ghosts of departed Quantities',[47] and further asserting that:

> Nothing is easier than to assign names, signs, or expressions to these fluxions; and it is not difficult to compute and to operate by means of such signs. But it will be found much more difficult to omit the signs and yet retain in our minds the things we suppose to be signified by them.[48]

For Berkeley, the term 'fluxion' is referent-blind, the equivalent of the term 'beautiful' for the blind man of Puiseaux, and describing himself as 'all in the dark', he asks those 'with the bright eyes' to show him a fluxion.[49]

Hobson and Harvey suggested that the *Analyst* controversy might be part of the backdrop to the *Letter*.[50] That would seem to be right; indeed, it may inform the *Letter*'s presentation of Saunderson. As Helena M. Pycior has shown in *Symbols, Impossible Numbers and Geometric Entanglements* (1997), though the real Saunderson took no part in the *Analyst* controversy itself, his *Elements of Algebra* subtly makes the case in favour of algebraic analysis, a case that Newton was not himself prepared to make in the aftermath of Berkeley's criticisms.[51] That is to say, Saunderson's *Elements* suggest the virtues of 'cogitatio cæca'. Pycior relates his defence of algebra to his physical blindness, claiming that it meant he had less use than the sighted for visual demonstrations,[52] which leads her to play down the role of his 'palpable arithmetic' in the *Elements*. Though she acknowledges its

---

46 See Helena M. Pycior, 'Mathematics and Philosophy: Wallis, Hobbes, Barrow and Berkeley'. *Journal of the History of Ideas*, 48 (1987), 265–286; Geoffrey Cantor, 'Berkeley's *Analyst* revisited'. *Isis* 75.4 (1984), 668–683.

47 George Berkeley, *The Analyst; or, A discourse addressed to an infidel mathematician: Wherein it is examined whether the object, principles, and inferences of the modern analysis are more distinctly conceived, or more evidently deduced, than religious mysteries and points of faith* (London: Printed for J. Tonson in the Strand, 1734), p. 59.

48 Berkeley, *The Analyst*, pp. 61–2.

49 George Berkeley, *A Defence of Free-Thinking in Mathematics in answer to a Pamphlet of Philalethes Cantabrigiensis, intituled, Geometry no Friend to Infidelity, or a Defence of Sir Isaac Newton, and the British Mathematicians* (London: Printed for J. Tonson in the Strand, 1735), p. 42. The metaphors of sight and blindness can also be found in Buffon's satirical account of Berkeley's intervention (see *Méthode des fluxions, et des suites infinies*, par M. le Chevalier Newton (Paris: chez De Bure l'aîné, Libraire, Quai des Augustins à Saint Paul, 1740), pp. xxv–xxvi).

50 Hobson and Harvey, p. 10 and p. 179, note 47.

51 Helena M. Pycior, *Symbols, Impossible Numbers and Geometric Entanglements* (Cambridge: Cambridge University Press, 1997), pp. 176–306.

52 Pycior, *Symbols, Impossible Numbers and Geometric Entanglements*, pp. 281–2.

presence, she argues that the overall aim of the work is to show that mathematical calculations can be performed without guidance from sensible figures, whether visible or palpable.[53] The contrast with the Saunderson of the *Letter* is significant; *** gives a very prominent role to the palpable arithmetic, presenting it as Saunderson's most important achievement. Why?

From Pycior's perspective, which is that of a historian of British mathematics, a defence of sensible demonstrations could only be reactionary, a concession to Berkeley and a backward step with respect to the scientific progress afforded by blind, symbolic reasoning. In the context of the mid eighteenth century in France, however, the claim that all knowledge was located in the senses and thus amenable to sensible demonstration was rich in heterodox implications, and *** takes the opportunity to suggest that even Newtonian mathematics is rooted in touch. It would no doubt be going too far to say that *** is suggesting that Saunderson could have made Berkeley touch the 'Ghost of a departed Quantity', but he does say, '[j]'ai lu avec toute l'attention dont je suis capable ce que Saunderson a dit de l'infini: je puis vous assurer qu'il avait sur ce sujet des idées très justes et très nettes, et que la plupart de nos infinitaires n'auraient été pour lui que des aveugles' [I read as attentively as I could what Saunderson had to say about infinity, and I can assure you that his ideas on that subject were very accurate and very clear, and that to him, most of our infinitesimalists would have been mere blind men].[54] In addition, *** is insistent that all mathematical reasoning must be based on sensory evidence; if Saunderson could lecture on optics, it is because, though the phenomena may be unavailable to him, the suppositions that underly his calculations are 'toutes relatives à des causes palpables' [all related to palpable causes].[55]

Yet just as we start feeling that human knowledge has a firm foundation we can touch, *** takes it away. He begins by exploring blindspots in applied maths, in which some of the figures in the calculations are necessarily estimates, and even if the results accurately describe the phenomenon, every single estimate could still be wrong.[56] Far more disconcerting than this, however, are the metaphysical principles that *** imagines would have been the basis for a Saundersonian work of geometry. *** acknowledges that Saunderson did not write such a work, but he claims that had he done so, it would have been based on highly abstract principles, close to those of the '*idéalistes*' [Idealists], who 'n'ayant conscience que de leur existence et des sensations qui se succèdent au

53 Pycior, *Symbols, Impossible Numbers and Geometric Entanglements*, pp. 282–3.
54 DPV, 4, p. 46; Hobson and Harvey, p. 57. *Letter*, p. 197.
55 DPV, 4, p. 42; Hobson and Harvey, p. 54; *Letter*, p. 195.
56 DPV, 4, p. 44; Hobson and Harvey, p. 56; *Letter*, p. 196.

dedans d'eux-mêmes, n'admettent pas autre chose' [are conscious only of their existence and of the sequence of sensations they experience inside themselves, and therefore admit nothing else].[57] This goes far beyond the earlier reference to the pure geometrical abstractions that had no empirical instanciation and were arrived at by the Supreme Being independently of any sensory experience; it refers instead to the claim that none of our ideas, whether of line or of colour, can be said to have a material object underlying it. While referent-blindness had earlier been overcome by referring symbols to ideas obtained from another sense, namely touch, *** now imagines ideas themselves, whether visual or haptic, to be referent-free, that is, unsupported by an external, material world.

Blind beliefs, as reported by ***, have thus gone from one heterodox extreme to the other: earlier the blind were said to be inclined to believe only matter to exist, and now Saunderson is imagined to hold the diametrically opposite view, namely that ideas alone exist. And just as the thinking-matter hypothesis was presented in a strikingly paradoxical manner and was followed by a sudden and spectacular change of both subject and register, so here no sooner does *** mention idealism than he condemns it in terms that are remarkable not least for their sudden reversal of the connotations of blindness. Up to this point, Saunderson's blindness had been shown in a positive light, but *** now describes the idealism to which he is imagined to have subscribed as '[un] système extravagant qui ne pouvait, ce me semble, devoir sa naissance qu'à des aveugles; système qui, à la honte de l'esprit humain et de la philosophie, est le plus difficile à combattre, quoique le plus absurde de tous' [an extravagant system which could only, it seems to me, have been born of the blind, a system which, to the shame of the human mind and philosophy, is the most difficult to refute, despite being the most absurd of all].[58] And *** makes explicit mention of Berkeley, accusing him of wilful blindness in the *Dialogues* that set out the Idealist system with 'autant de franchise que de clarté' [as much sincerity as clarity].[59] Yet whereas earlier, a similar reversal in the connotations of blindness signalled a clear shift in viewpoint away from atheism and the thinking-matter hypothesis to orthodox Christianity, here the viewpoint signalled by the volte-face is less clear: ***'s condemnation of idealism as blind could be voiced either from an orthodox standpoint of dualism or from a diametrically opposed

57 DPV, 4, p. 44; Hobson and Harvey, p. 56; *Letter*, p. 196.

58 DPV, 4, p. 44; Hobson and Harvey, p. 56; *Letter*, p. 196.

59 Bourdin simply dismisses the reference to Berkeley as confused and reductive (*Diderot. Le materialisme*, p. 42). For a study of the presence of Berkeley in Diderot's later writing, see my 'Eyes Wide Shut: *Le Rêve de d'Alembert*', in *New Essays on Diderot*, James Fowler (ed.) (Cambridge: Cambridge University Press, 2011), pp. 141–57.

standpoint, namely that of another heterodoxy, itself diametrically opposed to idealism, namely materialism. In the latter case, the *Letter* would be seen not only to stage the sighted opposing the blind, but also the blind opposing the blind.

Further opportunity to reflect on the position from which *** speaks and on how we might read what he says arises when *** explores the manner in which Saunderson spoke and in particular his use of 'felicitous expressions'.

Felicitous Expressions

We recall that the man-born-blind of Puiseaux spoke to the sighted as though he was sighted too, employing signs referent-free. Saunderson, by contrast, spoke to the sighted as though it were they who were blind. As a result, his speech was, so *** tells us, full of 'des expressions heureuses' [felicitous expressions]. The phrase is taken directly from Saunderson's 'Memoirs', where it appears merely in passing,[60] and so *** imagines what was meant: '[des expressions] qui sont propres à un sens, au toucher par exemple, et qui sont métaphoriques en même temps à un autre sens, comme aux yeux, d'où il résulte une double lumière pour celui à qui l'on parle, la lumière vraie et directe de l'expression, et la lumière réfléchie de la métaphore' [expressions that are appropriate to one sense, to touch for instance, and at the same time, metaphorical to another, such as sight, producing a dual light for the person being spoken to, the true and direct light of the expression, and the reflected light of the metaphor].[61] So where the man-born-blind of Puiseaux repeated what everyone else said, Saunderson didn't understand the half of what he was saying.[62]

Here, as earlier, however, before we settle in to feeling superior, *** explains that language is prone accidentally to escape the control of any speaker, whether blind or sighted: 'Cet accident est commun aux idiots qui font quelquefois d'excellentes plaisanteries, et aux personnes qui ont le plus d'esprit, à qui il échappe une sottise, sans que ni les uns ni les autres s'en aperçoivent' [Such a mishap is common to idiots who occasionally crack excellent jokes, and to the cleverest of people who sometimes let slip a stupid remark, and neither realize what they have said].[63] We are none of us, it would appear, any more than half aware of what it is we have said.

---

60 Saunderson, 'Memoirs', in *Elements*, vol. 1, p. iv.

61 DPV, 4, p. 41; Hobson and Harvey, p. 53; *Letter*, pp. 193–4. The adjective 'heureux' [felicitous] is also used to describe metaphorical language use in the *Encyclopédie* article 'Encyclopédie' by *, see vol. 5, p. 636.

62 We recall the man-born-blind-of-Puiseaux's remark about his ability to speak, which *** said contained more philosophy than he intended (above, p. 194).

63 DPV, 4, p. 41; Hobson and Harvey, p. 53; *Letter*, pp. 79–81.

There are, of course, implications for our reading of the *Letter*. *** is ironically suggesting that he too might be only half-aware of – and therefore only half-responsible for – what he has said; the other half is the reader's share. This is a standard topos of sceptical and freethinking writing. We might think of Bayle's imperative, 'Il faut laisser deviner au lecteur la moitié de ce qu'on veut dire pour le moins' [The reader must be left to work out at least half of what is meant],[64] which would be echoed by Voltaire in the *Dictionnaire philosophique* [Philosophical Dictionary] (1764): 'Les livres les plus utiles sont ceux dont les lecteurs font eux-mêmes la moitié.'[65] The implication is that if we see crime everywhere in the *Letter*, it's because we went looking for it.

Further implications for the *Letter* are suggested when *** explains that 'felicitous expressions' are not only the result of the speaker being blind to half the referents; they can also be caused by an entirely opposite phenomenon: a speaker can be rendered semi-mute owing either to a paucity of words or to a surfeit of ideas. This is the position, so *** tells Madame, in which both foreigners and writers find themselves, the former because they have more ideas than they know words, and the latter because they have more ideas than there are words to know. What he says of the writer is a variation on Marivaux's defence of (his own) style in *Le Cabinet du philosophe* [The Philosopher's Cabinet] (1734), in which Marivaux's philosopher explained that since words were the signs for ideas, a 'precious' style was not to be criticized; it was the sign of the speaker's subtle and original perceptions and ideas.[66] Sure enough the (half-hidden) reference to Marivaux soon emerges, along with that to Tacitus, which I also mentioned in the Introduction; *** explains that foreigners and writers are forced to adopt:

> des tours de phrases qui sont admirables toutes les fois qu'ils ne sont ni précieux ni obscurs, défauts qu'on leur pardonne plus ou moins difficilement, selon qu'on a plus d'esprit soi-même et moins de connaissance de la langue. Voilà pourquoi M. de M. . . est de tous les auteurs français, celui qui plaît le plus aux Anglais, et Tacite, celui de tous les auteurs latins que les *Penseurs* estiment davantage. Les

---

64 Pierre Bayle, *Œuvres diverses*, Elisabeth Labrousse (ed.), 9 volumes (Hildesheim: G. Olms, 1964–90), vol. 5.1, p. 144.

65 Voltaire, *Oeuvres complètes* (Oxford: Voltaire Foundation, 1968–), vol. 35, p. 284. Both Bayle and Voltaire's phrases might also be said to echo a statement in Montaigne: '[l]a parole est moitié à celuy qui parle, moitié à celuy qui l'escoute' [speech belongs half to the speaker and half to the listener]. (*Essais*, p. 1088; *Essays*, p. 1016).

66 Pierre Carlet de Chamblain de Marivaux, *Le Cabinet du philosophe* (Paris: Prault, 1734), p. 132.

> licences de langage nous échappent, et la vérité des termes nous frappe seule.[67]

> turns of phrase that are admirable as long as they are neither precious nor obscure, qualities we forgive more or less easily depending how much more wit and how much less knowledge of the language we have than they do. That is why, of all French writers, M. de M. . . is the one the English love most, and why Tacitus is the Latin writer whom *Thinkers* hold in the highest esteem. The linguistic liberties they take pass us by, and we are struck only by the truth of the terms.[68]

There are some tricksy moves here which need our attention. Initially, *** does not identify himself with either the English or the *Thinkers* – his French is better than that of the former, and his wit sharper than that of the typographically self-important latter. And yet in the final sentence, relationships are reconfigured by the first-person plural pronoun so that what had seemed to be linguistic incompetence on the part of the English and dim-wittedness on the part of the *Thinkers* becomes 'our' ability to appreciate Marivaux's witty constructions and Tacitus's verbal allusions. (Perhaps the italics and the capital letter of *Thinkers* signalled that it was the opposition's term of abuse?) And so where, earlier, we were required to supply half the meaning because the blind speaker didn't know the half of what he was saying, now we are required to supply half the words because the visionary writer can't say the half of what he thinks.

Again there are important implications for our reading: is *** inviting the reader to see and hear in those turns of phrase, which might appear almost precious or somewhat obscure, the signs of new, hitherto unspoken and perhaps unspeakable ideas? And if so, what are they? Can the reader give voice to them in ***'s place? Raphson's 'ingenious expression' suggests that atheism is one idea that can only be expressed in a semi-precious or *chiaroscuro* manner, and the same would seem to be true for the thinking-matter hypothesis given ***'s strikingly paradoxical formulation of it earlier.

Yet perhaps there does come a moment when a person can express his or her views sincerely and clearly – a moment just before death. We turn now to explore what Saunderson is supposed to have said on his deathbed.

---

67 DPV, 4, p. 42; Hobson and Harvey, p. 54 (this edition omits the capital letter and the italics of '*Penseurs*').

68 *Letter*, p. 194.

Five

A Supplement to Saunderson's 'Memoirs'

Retrospectively conveying a sense that much of the *Letter* had been building towards the account of Saunderson's last moments, *** now tells Madame, 'Mais ne nous éloignons plus de Saunderson, et suivons cet homme extraordinaire jusqu'au tombeau' [But let's move no further away from Saunderson and follow this extraordinary man to the grave]. The account of his last moments is, we recall, supposedly taken from a work written by one of Saunderson's 'disciples', a certain Mr William Inchliff, and entitled *The Life and Character of Nicholas Saunderson*. As we'll see, it can be read (or, rather, ***'s alleged translation of it can be read) as revealing there was something missing from the real Saunderson's 'Memoirs' and supplying it.

An Omission

The real 'Memoirs' say that Saunderson had no interest in metaphysics because it 'dealt in such abstract ideas as have not the objects of sense for their foundation',[1] a claim that contrasts (or which the *Letter* makes contrast with) the claim that the blind are 'more abstracted' than the sighted. That claim is, of course, potentially ambiguous: if we take metaphysics to incude theology, his lack of interest in it could be taken to mean that he was an unbeliever. Nothing else indicates as much in the 'Memoirs', however, and his death is recounted as follows:

> [Saunderson] received this notice of his approaching death with great calmness and serenity; and after a short silence, resumed life and spirits, and talked with as much composure of mind as he had ever done in the most sedate hours of perfect health. He appointed the evening of the following day to receive the sacrament with Mr. Holmes; but before that came, he was seized with a delirium, which continued to his death.[2]

1 Saunderson, 'Memoirs' in *Elements*, vol. 1, p. iii.
2 Saunderson, 'Memoirs' in *Elements*, vol. 1, p. xix.

Yet dying without receiving the sacrament does seem to have aroused suspicion. The *Biographia Britannica* (1765) contains an entry on Saunderson, in which it is stated that:

> He received the notice of his approaching death with great calmness and serenity; and, after a short silence, resuming life and spirit, he talked with as much composure as usual. He was supposed not to entertain any great notion of revealed religion; yet we are told, he appointed to receive the sacrament the evening before his death, which a delirium that never went off, prevented him from doing.[3]

The two corrective clauses of the second sentence are suggestive: 'yet we are told' undermines the earlier report that Saunderson was 'supposed not to entertain any great notion of revealed religion', but it is itself undermined by subsequent and rather neat coincidence, given his supposed lack of religious notions, of Saunderson's earlier-than-predicted death, which meant that he did not receive the sacraments (after all?). (It is the same kind of looping-back logic that we encountered in the opening paragraph of the *Letter*: *** didn't want to see Réaumur's experiment, but he agreed to nevertheless, and then Réaumur stopped him seeing it.) By the nineteenth century, the suggestion that he might have been an unbeliever seems to have become a remarkable certainty. George Dyer reports as follows in *The Privileges of the University of Cambridge* (1824):

> [Whiston] being deprived for some religious opinions, and Saunderson being no friend to divine revelation – in like manner as Dr. Halley, Professor of Astronomy at Oxford, Saunderson's contemporary – it was remarked, that as Whiston was set aside on account of too much religion, Saunderson was preferred for having none at all. Saunderson's talents and attainments, however, did, in the judgement of Sir Isaac Newton himself, eminently qualify him for the professor's chair, whatever he might think on religious matters; and he was much admired for his regard to veracity both in profession and practice. It is remarkable, that though Saunderson was known to be an unbeliever, he desired to receive the communion before he died, which reminds us of Socrates's last request.[4]

---

3 *Biographia Britannica*, supplement, vol 7 (1765), pp. 157–8; see also Hobson and Harvey, p. 219. Hobson and Harvey observe that no explicit conclusion is drawn, but they draw none either.

4 George Dyer, *The Privileges of the University of Cambridge*, 2 volumes (London: Longman, 1824), vol. 2, p. 143.

Edmond Halley was known to be an atheist; indeed, the 'infidel mathematician' to whom Berkeley addressed his *Analyst* (1730) has often been thought to be Halley, following the story that he was responsible for the physician, Samuel Garth, refusing the last rites.[5] And as for Socrates' last request that a cock be given to the God, Asclepius, it is famously puzzling, given Socrates's denial of the existence of the Athenian gods: was it serious or ironic? Dyer clearly read it as ironic and thought Saunderson's request for the last rites was too.

Diderot seems to have read the 'Memoirs' in a similarly suspicious manner. He has Inchlif report in the invented *Life and Character*, supposedly quoted by *** in translation in the *Letter*, a number of arguments against the existence of God that Saunderson put to his vicar, Holmes, who had perhaps come to administer the last sacraments.[6] With respect to the 'Memoirs', Inchlif supplies what the 'Memoirs' seems to have omitted, namely what it was that Saunderson said before he died. Yet when he argued against God's existence, was he speaking with 'as much composure of mind as he ever had done in the most sedate hours of perfect health' or was he in a 'delirium'?

A Conversation about the Existence of God

Many of the ideas and arguments that appear in the conversation between Holmes and Saunderson about the existence of God have already appeared in embryonic form earlier in the *Letter*. What Saunderson says to Holmes echoes what *** thought a blind man might think, and as a result, Holmes's responses to Saunderson appear to the reader as a series of rather short-sighted gaffes.

We do not hear exactly how Saunderson began the conversation – the *in medias res* technique contributes to the fiction of the fragmentary nature of the surviving record. Not only does this put Holmes in the position of making a counter-argument, as though Saunderson's view was the established one, but the argument he makes does not bode well: he appeals to 'les merveilles de la nature' [nature's marvels].[7] Earlier, *** had already observed that the blind found that argument 'very weak', and predictably, Saunderson agrees: 'laissez là tout ce beau spectacle qui n'a jamais été fait pour moi! J'ai été condamné à passer ma vie dans les ténèbres, et vous me citez des prodiges que je n'entends point, et qui ne prouvent que pour

5 Geoffrey Cantor has suggested that such a reading of *The Analyst*, though common, is too restrictive, and it is better understood to be directed at all deists and freethinkers in general (see 'Berkeley's *The Analyst* revisited'. *Isis*, 75 (1984), 668–83).

6 Though it was not translated into English until 1770 (see below, p. 167), it is not impossible that the *Letter* influenced the *Biographia Britannia*'s claim that Saunderson was 'no friend to revealed religion'.

7 DPV, 4, p. 48; Hobson and Harvey, p. 59; *Letter*, p. 199.

vous et que pour ceux qui voient comme vous' [forget that beautiful great spectacle that was never made for me! I have been condemned to live my life in darkness, and you cite wonders I can't understand and which are proof only for you and those who see as you do].[8] Holmes has come up with an argument that not only gives Saunderson a rather painful reminder of his disability, which he views in terms of condemnation, and for which a blind man can access no empirical evidence, though ironically he uses a metaphor of deafness ('je n'entends point') to convey how incomprehensible he finds it.

What the blind man says he needs is some empirical evidence in a form he can comprehend, namely touch, and so Holmes asks him to run his hands over his body, to which he refers, using the vocabulary of the argument from design, as a 'mécanisme' [mechanism].[9] To the reader, however, this has all the makings of another blunder. Although it recalls ***'s earlier claim about the blind man being able to sense by his touch 'how the parts of a whole have to be arranged such that we call it beautiful', *** had also observed that the haptic idea of beauty was restricted to utility: '[l]a beauté, pour un aveugle n'est qu'un mot, quand elle est séparée de l'utilité' [to a blind man, beauty is nothing more than a word when it is separated from utility].[10] Here not only is the body that Saunderson perceives not as beautiful to his touch as it is to Holmes's sight but, since the eyes don't work, it's not as useful either. Things are not going well for the deist vicar.

However, as Lorraine Daston and Katherine Park have shown in their *Wonders and the Order of Nature, 1150–1750* (1998), the standard theological view of disfigurements and deformities was that they were, precisely, signs or wonders, evidence of divine power, as the etymological link between 'monster' and 'monstrare' [to show] makes clear.[11] If Saunderson is to argue his case effectively, he might have to counter that view of blindness and, as Andrew Curran has shown, his argument does indeed make complex and sometimes contradictory use of the conception of blindness as a sign.[12] Saunderson goes on to acknowledge to Holmes that other people have indeed seen him as an object of wonder, but then explains that this is shortsighted of them:

> J'ai été si souvent un objet d'admiration pour vous, que j'ai bien mauvaise opinion de ce qui vous surprend. J'ai attiré du fond de

---

8 DPV, 4, p. 48; Hobson and Harvey, p. 59; *Letter*, p. 199.

9 DPV, 4, p. 48; Hobson and Harvey, p. 59; *Letter*, p. 199.

10 DPV, 4, p. 19; Hobson and Harvey, p. 30; *Letter*, p. 172.

11 Lorraine Daston and Katherine Park, *Wonders and the Order of Nature, 1150–1750* (Cambridge, MA: MIT Press, 1998).

12 Curran, *Sublime Disorder*, pp. 58–79.

> l'Angleterre des gens qui ne pouvaient concevoir comment je faisais de la géométrie: il faut que vous conveniez que ces gens-là n'avaient pas de notions bien exactes de la possibilité des choses.[13]

> I have been the object of your wonder so often that I have a very low opinion of the things that amaze you. People have come to see me from all over England because they could not imagine how I was able to do geometry, which you must admit means that such people did not have a very clear notion of what is possible.[14]

He will later evoke the infinite possibilities of the universe, but here he adopts a moralist's position, attacking human vanity, a fault often described, of course, as blind: 'Un phénomène est-il, à notre avis, au-dessus de l'homme, nous disons aussitôt, c'est l'ouvrage d'un Dieu; notre vanité ne se contente pas à moins: ne pourrions-nous pas mettre dans nos discours un peu moins d'orgueil et un peu plus de philosophie?' [If we think a phenomenon is beyond man, we immediately say it's God's work; our vanity will accept nothing less, but couldn't we be a bit less vain and a bit more philosophical in what we say?].[15] And making use of his simple mode of reasoning, he appeals to the principle of Ockham's razor:

> Si la nature nous offre un noeud difficile à délier, laissons-le pour ce qu'il est, et n'employons pas à le couper la main d'un être qui devient ensuite pour nous un nouveau noeud plus indissoluble que le premier. Demandez à un Indien pourquoi le monde reste suspendu dans les airs, il vous répondra qu'il est porté sur le dos d'un éléphant, et l'éléphant sur quoi l'appuiera-t-il? Sur une tortue; et la tortue, qui la soutiendra? . . . Cet Indien vous fait pitié, et l'on pourrait vous dire comme à lui: Monsieur Holmes mon ami, confessez d'abord votre ignorance, et faites-moi grâce de l'éléphant et de la tortue.[16]

> If nature presents us with a problem that is difficult to unravel, let's leave it as it is and not try to undo it with the help of a being who then offers us a new problem, more insoluble than the first. Ask an Indian how the world stays up in the air, and he'll tell you that an elephant is carrying it on its back; and the elephant, what's he standing on? A tortoise. And that tortoise, what's keeping him up? . . . To you, that Indian is pitiful, yet one could say the same of you

13 DPV, 4, p. 49; Hobson and Harvey, p. 60.
14 *Letter*, p. 199.
15 DPV, 4, p. 49; Hobson and Harvey, p. 60; *Letter*, pp. 199–200.
16 DPV, 4, p. 48; Hobson and Harvey, p. 60.

> as you say of him. So, Mr Holmes, my friend, start by confessing your ignorance, and let's do without the elephant and the tortoise.[17]

The tables are turned on Holmes here: it is not the dying blind man who should confess, but his sighted minister, and it is not his sins he should be confessing, but his ignorance. The reference to 'Indian' philosophy is worth noting. While Colas Duflo is right to say that in the *Entretiens sur la pluralité des mondes*, Fontenelle refers to an 'Indian' philosopher who claims that the world is held in space because it is balanced on the back of elephants, the tortoises are not Diderot's invention.[18] They come instead from Locke's *Essay* and they appear in a discussion, not of space but of substance. Locke compares the 'Indian' view of space, according to which the world stands on an elephant who, in turn, stands on a 'broad-back'd Tortoise',[19] to our supposition that a material substance underlies the sensible qualities we perceive, a supposition he presents as both as absurd as the 'Indian' view and as a perfectly acceptable working hypothesis.[20] It is, of course, the materialist implications of that hypothesis that Berkeley rejects when he replaces matter by God (though, for obvious reasons, he does so with no mention of elephants and tortoises). In the *Letter*, by a comic process of slippage, elephants and tortoises no longer stand for space nor for material substance, but for God, and to Saunderson, that hypothesis is unworkable.

All Holmes can do now is appeal to authority. He cites Newton, Leibniz and Clarke, calling them 'les premiers génies du monde' [the world's foremost geniuses],[21] and reminds Saunderson that they could not only see the beautiful design of the universe but they also attributed it to a divine designer. Indeed, Bergier would later observe in *Deism refuted* that since a blind man does not deny the existence of colour just because he cannot see it, atheism cannot draw any strength from the blind man's inability to see design in the world. However, for the reader of the *Letter*, this is to ask Saunderson to behave like three-quarters of ***'s theatre-goers who simply rely on other people's judgements. It is then perhaps rather surprising to hear Saunderson accede to Holmes's request that he believe in authority. He does so, however, only as a momentary concession in a much bigger strategy.

---

17 *Letter*, p. 200.

18 Duflo, *Diderot philosophe*, p. 106. Maillet's work of natural history, *Telliamed*, is also supposed to be a conversation between an Indian philosopher and a French missionary.

19 Locke, *Essay*, p. 296; see also p. 175.

20 Jonathan Bennett has written of 'the doubleness of attitude' in the passages about substance in Locke's *Essay*; see 'Substratum'. *History of Philosophy Quarterly*, 4.2 (1987), 197–215, p. 197.

21 DPV, 4, p. 49; Hobson and Harvey, p. 60; *Letter*, p. 200.

The blind man offers his minister a deal: he will accept the evidence of authority with respect to the current order, visible to others in the universe, in exchange for the freedom to think what he pleases about its origins, and he takes some pleasure in observing to Holmes that in that regard, '[V]ous n'êtes pas moins aveugle que moi. Vous n'avez point ici de témoins à m'opposer, et vos yeux ne vous sont d'aucune resource' [You are no less blind than I am. You have no witnesses here to testify against me, and your eyes are of no use to you].[22] We never hear whether Holmes accepts the deal since he makes no further contributions to the conversation or, at least, no further verbal ones – later he will burst into tears. And what Saunderson 'sees' challenges the idea that the current state of things, admirably ordered though it may be, could be either the result of a guiding intelligence or in any way stable and permanent. Saunderson replaces the perpetually geometrizing God with matter in perpetual and random motion, and he does so in part on the evidence of his own body.

An Epicurean 'Vision'

As numerous critics have persuasively shown, Saunderson presents an Epicurean vision of the origins and working of the universe that draws on Lucretius's poem, *De Rerum Natura*, in a manner similar to the emerging (though often clandestinely published) discourses of natural history to which we referred earlier. The ancient poem was the subject of much critical debate in the first half of the eighteenth century, notably in the years surrounding the publication of the *Letter* when, for example, Polignac published his *Anti-Lucretius* (1747),[23] and Lelarge de Lignac would subsequently dub Buffon's *Histoire naturelle* 'Anti-Polignac'.[24] Saunderson's vision can be seen as another intervention within this controversy.

We might wonder why it is that a blind man is made to voice an Epicurean vision of the workings of nature in the *Letter*. Jean-Claude Bourdin's view is that Saunderson's blindness allows Diderot to underscore the hypothetical, conjectural status of his materialism that is without a secure basis in empirical science.[25] Saunderson does indeed often draw attention to the fact that his claims do not rely on empirical evidence, declaring: 'je conjecture donc' [It is therefore my conjecture].[26] There is more to it than this, however; to have a blind man articulate a specifically

22 DPV, 4, p. 50; Hobson and Harvey, p. 61; *Letter*, p. 200.

23 See Melchior de Polignac, *Anti-Lucretius, sive De Deo et natura, libri novem* (Paris: Henri-Louis Guerin and Jean Guerin, 1747).

24 Joseph Adrien Lelarge de Lignac, *Lettres à un Américain sur l'histoire naturelle, générale et particulière de Monsieur de Buffon*, 5 volumes (Hamburg: n.p., 1751), vol. 1, p. 4.

25 Bourdin, *Diderot*, pp. 51–52.

26 DPV, 4, p. 51; Hobson and Harvey, p. 62; *Letter*, p. 201.

Epicurean vision of the universe involves literalizing a metaphor that was commonly used to describe it: Epicurean nature was often said to be, precisely, 'blind'.

We read, for example, in Hume's *Enquiry concerning Human Understanding* (1748) of 'chance, or blind and unguided force of matter',[27] and many similar examples could be offered in both English and French – the *Encyclopédie*, for instance, contains many examples of this usage.[28] What is noteworthy is the frequently polemical force of the term 'blind'. Hume's text makes this clear: although the phrase is spoken by an Epicurean, he is paraphrasing the arguments of his 'accusers'. He says: 'there appear such marks of intelligence and design [in the order of nature], that you think it extravagant to assign for its cause, either chance, or the blind and unguided force of matter.'[29]

Whether ascribed to nature, matter or chance, 'blind' is almost always a charge made against the Epicureans by the opposing side, relying on the negative connotations of blindness.[30] This may perhaps account for the fact that while Saunderson clearly envisages nature as blind, he does not himself use the adjective to describe the natural processes he envisages. The parallel between a blind man's view of blind nature is left to the reader to draw, and depending on her point of view, the fact that a blind man is an Epicurean either successfully appropriates the term in advance of the opposition in a kind of pre-emptive strike or suggests that his metaphysical point of view is merely relative to and perhaps even determined by his bodily organization. What is certain, however, is that Saunderson will use his own blindness as evidence against his opponent; he will be the prime witness in his own case against God.

He asks Holmes to suppose that in the beginning, there was no seven-day divine master plan. Instead, he is to suppose that matter moved on its own and molecules came together to form organisms, most of which were

---

27 David Hume, An *Enquiry concerning Human Understanding*, Peter Millican (ed.) (Oxford: Oxford University Press, 2007), p. 99.

28 In the *Encyclopédie*, the term 'blind' qualifies nature as envisaged by Epicurus (see article 'Création'), by Spinoza (see article 'Ame' [Soul]), and by the Cambridge Platonists, More and Cudworth, whose 'plastic nature' was thought by many to be close to that of Spinoza (see article 'Plastique').

29 Hume, *Enquiry*, p. 99.

30 The anonymous *Dissertation sur la formation du monde* [Dissertation on the formation of the world] (1738) contains a rare example of the term being used without pejorative connotations; it speaks of the world as a 'chef d'œuvre d'un architecte aveugle, l'exacte géométrie en était bannie' [a blind architect's masterpiece from which geometrical recision had been banished]. (*Dissertation sur la formation du monde (1738); Dissertation sur la résurrection de la chair (1743): manuscrits du recueil 1168 de la Bibliothèque Mazarine de Paris*, Claudia Stancati (ed.) (Paris: Champion, 2001), p. 123).

not even viable, let alone beautiful or symmetrical. Having just agreed to accept the mathematicians' vision of the present order of the world, he challenges their view of the past: 'qui vous a dit à vous, à Leibniz, à Clarke et à Newton, que dans les premiers instants de la formation des animaux, les uns n'étaient pas sans tête et les autres sans pieds?] [who told you all, you, Leibniz, Clarke and Newton, that when animals first came into being, there weren't some with no heads and others with no feet?].[31] Like Lucretius, Saunderson imagines all kinds of freaks and monsters, most of whom would have failed to live very long because they lacked not only heads or feet, but also stomachs or intestines, or they had heart or lung defects instead, or they had defective reproductive organs, or they never met a mate.[32] On this Lucretian view, the survival of the human race is not so much a successful outcome of random collisions as the least defective outcome.[33] Indeed, man could very easily never have come about at all; he might have been and perhaps forever have remained 'au nombre des possibles' [one of a number of possible outcomes].[34] It is now that Saunderson decides to follow Holmes's advice and consider his own body, but he draws from it precisely the opposite conclusion: Saunderson identifies himself as one of Lucretius's freaks. He says manipulatively, 'Voyez-moi bien, Monsieur Holmes, je n'ai point d'yeux' [Look me in the face, Mr Holmes; I have no eyes].[35] Saunderson's body proves Lucretius right: he is a sign, after all, but one that demonstrates the accuracy of the Epicurean vision.

Suddenly moving away from the Latin scientific poetry, however, Saunderson goes to meet Holmes on his own territory. Provocatively he asks, 'Qu'avions-nous fait à Dieu, vous et moi, un pour avoir cet organe, l'autre pour en être privé?' [What have we done to God, you and I, such that one of us has that organ, and the other is deprived of it?].[36] His question echoes the one the disciples asked Jesus about a man-born-blind: 'who did sin, this man, or his parents, that he was born blind?'[37] Yet not only does Saunderson ask it for himself to God's representative,

31 DPV, 4, p. 50; Hobson and Harvey, p. 61; *Letter*, p. 201.

32 Lucretius, *On the Nature of the Universe*, pp. 160–1 (book 4, lines 835–60).

33 Saunderson's claim that monsters 'vanished over time' has sometimes led critics to claim that this is an early version of the theory of evolution. However, Jacques Roger is right to say: 'I would like to state here once and for all that it is absolutely impossible to see in this text an early anticipation of Darwin's theory of natural selection [. . .] There is certainly a philosophical kinship between the two doctrines. But having been a disciple of Lucretius does not suffice to make one a precursor of Darwin's.' (*The Life Sciences in Eighteenth-Century French Thought*, p. 652, n. 66.)

34 DPV, 4, p. 51; Hobson and Harvey, p. 62; *Letter*, p. 201.

35 DPV, 4, p. 51; Hobson and Harvey, p. 62; *Letter*, p. 201.

36 DPV, 4, p. 51; Hobson and Harvey, p. 62; *Letter*, p. 201.

37 John 9.2.

but where Jesus replied to his disciples, 'Neither hath this man sinned, nor his parents: but that the works of God should be made manifest in him',[38] Holmes just bursts into tears (something, moreover, which the eyeless Saunderson is presumably unable to do). Monstrosity certainly demonstrates, but what it is made to show (up) here is the lamentable insufficiency of the argument from design.

Saunderson can now develop his Epicurean case in further detail, making the same claim about the world as he had done about man, namely that it is simply a possible outcome of the random combinations of matter.[39] If this world is indeed symmetrical and ordered, as Newton and Leibniz claimed, and indeed as Saunderson has, on their word, accepted it to be, its order and symmetry are random and will not last. The world is 'Un composé sujet à des révolutions qui toutes indiquent une tendance continuelle à la destruction; une succession rapide d'êtres qui s'entre-suivent, se poussent et disparaissent: une symétrie passagère; un ordre momentané' [A composite, subject to cycles of change, all of which exhibit a tendency towards destruction; a rapid series of beings that appear one after another, one replacing the next before vanishing; symmetry is fleeting, and order momentary].[40] There is no perpetual geometer, no cosmic order or divine symmetry; order and symmetry are things that humans impose on the world when they tidy the house and use a mirror. And if we think the order we see is permanent, it is only because we have lost sight of the merely transitory nature of our own lives, a fact of which the dying Saunderson is, no doubt, acutely aware: 'Le monde est éternel pour vous, comme vous êtes éternel pour l'être qui ne vit qu'un instant . . . Le temps, la matière et l'espace ne sont peut-être qu'un point' [The world is eternal to you, just as you are eternal to the being that only lives for an instant . . . Time, matter and space may be only a single dot].[41]

It is on that note that Saunderson became more agitated than his state of health would permit and, as though his own consciousness closes down into a single point, he entered a delirium. A reader who already knew the 'Memoirs' might have thought he had entered that delirium already; instead she now discovers that, in fact, this was him speaking 'with as much composure of mind as he had ever done in the most sedate hours of perfect health'. That same reader will also be expecting the delirium to last until his death. However, Inchlif's Saunderson emerges from it, and

---

38 John 9.3. We should note that Jesus continues: 'I must work the works of him that sent me, while it is day: the night cometh, when no man can work', and that *** reports that the man-born-blind of Puiseaux works, precisely, at night (DPV, 4, p. 18; Hobson and Harvey, p. 30; *Letter*, p. 172).

39 Lucretius, *On the Nature of the Universe*, p. 66 (book 2, lines 1060–70).

40 DPV, 4, p. 52; Hobson and Harvey, pp. 62–3; *Letter*, p. 202.

41 DPV, 4, p. 52; Hobson and Harvey, p. 63; *Letter*, p. 202.

in that supplementary moment of life, he utters some rather surprising final words.

Last Words

Inchlif reports that 'il lui survint un accès de délire qui dura quelques heures, et dont il ne sortit que pour s'écrier "*Ô Dieu de Clarke et de Newton, prends pitié de moi!*" et mourir' [he went into a delirium lasting several hours, from which he only emerged to exclaim, 'Oh God of Clarke and of Newton, take pity on me!' and die].[42] Saunderson's last words appear in italics perhaps to ensure that the 'people who see crime everywhere' have their eyes drawn to them and are reassured, but they should also draw our attention too. While many critics have overlooked them or disregarded them as ironic, it is more fruitful to identify and engage with the interpretive puzzles they offer.

Perhaps the first is, quite simply, why Diderot invented a supplement in which Saunderson confesses at all, let alone in the strange way that he does (to which we shall return in a moment). If the aim was to 'out' the real Saunderson as an atheist, then the real 'Memoirs' which say he died without the final sacraments would seem to provide a sufficient alibi for having him die unrepentant in the *Letter*. Moreover, there was a tradition of mathematicians refusing to confess on their deathbeds: it was widely reported that a dying Prince Maurice of Nassau (d. 1625) told his priest 'je crois que deux et deux font quatre',[43] a phrase that was guaranteed an afterlife when placed in the mouth of the freethinking hero of Molière's *Don Juan* (1665).[44] This tradition and the 'Memoirs' might seem to dispense with the need to have Saunderson make any confession at all. On the other hand, if the aim was to ensure that Saunderson's religious belief is heard, it might be thought that Diderot would have avoided a deathbed confession following La Mettrie's response to one of his previous publications. In *L'Homme machine*, La Mettrie had claimed that the *Pensées philosophiques* provided no better argument in favour of the existence of God than an atheist confessing on his deathbed, which he viewed as frivolous:

> Voyez, disent [les Déistes], les Spinoza, les Vanini, les Desbarreaux et les Boindin, apôtres qui font plus d'honneur, que de tort au déisme! La durée de la santé des ces derniers a été la mesure de

---

42 DPV, 4, p. 52; Hobson and Harvey, p. 63; *Letter*, p. 202.

43 Jean Louis Guez, seigneur de Balzac, *Socrate chrétien*, in *Œuvres*, L. Moreau (ed.), 2 volumes (Paris: J. Lecoffre, 1854), vol. 2, pp. 95–6. See also Tallement des Réaux, *Historiettes*, Antoine Adam (ed.), 2 volumes (Paris: Gallimard, 1960–61), vol. 1, p. 226.

44 Molière, *Don Juan*, in *Œuvres completes*, Georges Forestier (ed.), 2 volumes (Paris: Gallimard, 2010), vol. 2, p. 875.

> leur incrédulité: et il est rare en effet, ajoutent-ils, qu'on n'abjure pas l'athéisme, dès que les passions se sont affaiblies avec le corps qui en est l'instrument.
>
> Voilà certainement tout ce qu'on peut dire de plus favorable à l'existence d'un Dieu, quoique le dernier argument soit frivole, en ce que ces conversions sont courtes, l'esprit reprenant presque toujours ses anciennes opinions, et se conduisant en conséquence, dès qu'il a recouvré, ou plutôt retrouvé ses forces dans celles du corps. En voilà du moins beaucoup plus que n'en dit le médecin *Diderot*, dans ses *Pensées Philosophiques*, sublime ouvrage qui ne convaincra pas un athée.[45]

> Look, [the Deists] say, at the Spinozas, Vaninis, Desbarreaux and Boindins, apostles who do more to honour than harm Deism! Their unbelief only lasted as long as their health did, and they add that it is rare for people not to renounce atheism as soon as their passions have weakened with the body that is their instrument.
>
> That is certainly the most that can be said in favour of the existence of a God, although the last is a trifling argument, as such conversions are short-lived; the mind almost always returns to its former opinions and acts in consequence as soon as it recovers or rather renews its strength in that of the body. Anyway it is a lot more than is said by Doctor[46] Diderot in his *Philosophical Thoughts*, a sublime work, which will not convince an atheist.[47]

Inasmuch as the most Saunderson says in favour of the existence of God is, precisely, his dying words, is the *Letter* playfully engaging with La Mettrie's criticism of the *Pensées*?[48]

So, how are we to take Saunderson's dying words? This might be the moment to recall the earlier discussion of the phatic function of language to suggest that Saunderson simply utters these words in the same way as the man-born-blind of Puiseaux and three-quarters of theatre-goers declare plays to be beautiful: they fulfil a purely social obligation. Without wishing to identify Saunderson with Diderot, the latter was known to

---

45 Julien Offray de La Mettrie, *L'Homme Machine: A Study in the Origins of an Idea*, Aram Vartanian (ed.) (Princeton: Princeton University Press, 1960), p. 177.

46 Diderot was, of course, not a doctor, but he had translated Robert James's *Medical Dictionary*, which may have given La Mettrie this impression.

47 La Mettrie, *Machine Man and other writings*, Ann Thomson (ed.) (Cambridge: Cambridge University Press, 1996), p. 24 (translation slightly modified).

48 The *Pensées* is often read as the work of a deist. Yet La Mettrie's claim that its deism is not wholly convincing has truth to it and may indicate a deliberate strategy on Diderot's part, which is not dissimilar to that found in Saunderson's final words.

claim in the late 1740s that on his deathbed he would '[faire] comme les autres, qu'il se confessera et qu'il recevra ce que nous appellons notre Dieu, et s'il le fait ce ne sera point par devoir, que ce ne sera que par rapport à sa famille, de crainte qu'on ne leur reproche qu'il est mort de cette façon-là' [behave like everyone else, confess and receive what we call our God, and if he did so, it would not be out of duty, but for his family out of fear that they be reproached for the manner of his death].[49] Yet Saunderson's words are not purely phatic; they do have referential content or, rather, he does not quote the standard line.

Saunderson makes his final plea to a very specific God, that of Clarke and Newton. Moreover, in the context of the *Letter*, he appeals to precisely the eternal geometer whose existence his Epicurean vision of nature has just undermined. Furthermore, it is most peculiar to request pity from Clarke and Newton's God: he doesn't do pity (or love or grace etc.); he just blindly does his geometry. Moreover, were he merely blind, he would be able to hear Saunderson's plea, but the Supreme Being who thinks in pure abstractions is is completely insensible. Riskin's claim about solipsism is perhaps relevant here,[50] though it is not blind men who are indifferent to others' pain, but God.

Inchlif has nothing further to report of Saunderson's life and death, but *** is ready to pass judgement and what he says, while we could flatly dismiss it as ironic too, opens up more questions. Commenting on what he is supposed to have just translated, *** suggests that Saunderson was in need of some reassurance: 'Vous voyez, Madame, que tous les raisonnements qu'il venait d'objecter au ministre n'étaient pas même capables de rassurer un aveugle' [You see, Madame, even all those arguments that he had just put forward to the minister were not enough to reassure a blind man].[51] This idea of a need for reassurance is important and puzzling.

While ***'s words might be a nod to La Mettrie, who had said that deathbed confessions were unconvincing, they also suggest that Saunderson's Epicurean vision, perhaps that last part in particular, in which he saw himself as merely a tiny dot, was scary to him, nightmarish even. Andrew Curran has suggested that Saunderson had a post-modern prophecy, a vision of 'the frightening and bleak implications of so-called Enlightenment method',[52] and he is not the only critic to read Diderot as a proto-post-modern writer.[53] Yet Saunderson might instead have felt a different sort of fear: his final vision of himself as a tiny dot recalls that of man's 'disproportion' in the universe, which induced a feeling of 'effroi'

49 Quoted in Diderot's police file, see 'Diderot à Vincennes', p. 202.

50 See above, p. 74.

51 DPV, 4, p. 52; Hobson and Harvey, p. 63; *Letter*, p. 202.

52 Curran, *Sublime Disorder*, p. 79.

53 See Brewer, *The Discourse of Enlightenment*.

[terror] in the freethinker of Pascal's *Pensées*.[54] Saunderson's words to Holmes, telling him to go beyond what he can see, might be read as an ironic version of Pascal's desire to take the deist beyond what he can see.[55] Of course, where Pascal's aim was to show the deist that he was unable to see God, Saunderson's aim was to make Holmes see that if God was nowhere to be seen, it was because he did not exist. And yet Saunderson's subsequent need for reassurance suggests his strategy might have backfired: what he discovered was that Pascal was right not only because God is indeed, *pace* Holmes, nowhere to be seen and faith can only be blind, but also because in the giant abyss that lies beyond what we can see, only faith can provide any reassurance.

However, Saunderson's expression of that faith can also be read as twisting the Pascalian position back on itself. The blind man's last words are a reverse echo of Pascal's apostrophe, 'Dieu d'Abraham, Dieu d'Isaac, Dieu de Jacob, non des philosophes et des savants' [God of Abraham, God of Isaac, God of Jacob, not of philosophers and scholars].[56] Saunderson seems to have got things back to front: in need of some reassurance, he asks for pity not from Abraham, Isaac and Jacob's God but from the philosophers and scholars' geometer-God, a request all the more bizarre given that Abraham, Isaac and Jacob's God is by his very nature 'caché' [hidden] and thus more appropriate for the blind.[57] ***'s diagnosis of Saunderson's final words as a need for reassurance thus appears most peculiar.

Things only become more complicated as *** exclaims, 'Quelle honte pour des gens qui n'ont pas de meilleures raisons que lui, qui voient, et à qui le spectacle étonnant de la nature annonce, depuis le lever du soleil jusqu'au coucher des moindres étoiles, l'existence et la gloire de son auteur!' [It puts to shame those people whose arguments are no stronger than his, but who are able to see and to whom the amazing spectacle of nature, from the rising of the sun to the setting of the tiniest stars, proclaims the existence and glory of its author!].[58] We have heard

---

54 Blaise Pascal, *Œuvres complètes*, Louis Lafuma (ed.) (Paris: Editions du Seuil, 1963), fragments 198–9 [*Pensées and Other Writings*, Honor Levi (trans.), Anthony Levi (intro. and notes) (Oxford: Oxford World's Classics, 2008), fragment 230]. References to the French edition will be given by the fragment number preceded by the letter L; references to the English translation, which uses the Sellier classification of the 'Pensées', will be given by the fragment number preceded by the letter S. For a different reading of the role of Pascal in the *Letter*, see Duflo, *Diderot philosophe*, p. 122.

55 Pascal says he wishes to make microscopists, for example, see that what they see as a wonder of nature is, in fact, 'un abîme nouveau' [another abyss], L199 [S230].

56 L913 [S742].

57 L228 [S260].

58 DPV, 4, p. 52; Hobson and Harvey, p. 63; *Letter*, p. 202.

this exclamatory voice before, and we recall that his earlier exclamations were often subsequently undermined. Our eyes are peeled, and sure enough, the view expressed in the exclamation is almost immediately undercut. *** continues, 'Ils ont des yeux dont Saunderson était privé; mais Saunderson avait une pureté de moeurs et une ingénuité de caractère qui leur manquent. Aussi ils vivent en aveugles, et Saunderson meurt, comme s'il eût vu' [They have eyes, which Saunderson did not, and yet he had a purity of morals and an innocence of character that they lack. Thus they live their lives blind, and Saunderson dies as though he could see].[59] The logic is deliberately odd: because he saw the light at the end, Saunderson is compared favourably to the atheists, who are blind to the light despite being able to see, but the comparison is also favourable because of the way Saunderson lived, virtuously and honestly, while the atheists lack moral sense and are morally blind. This suggests that, in relation to the practice of virtue at least, religious faith is redundant: if the light only came to Saunderson in a final flash at the end, but he lived virtuously while throughout his life holding the views he expressed to Holmes, then a blind man, that is to say, an atheist, can live virtuously. Just because plenty do not, that does not mean it is not possible – Saunderson even asked Holmes not to cry over his death in order to ensure he had never in his life been guilty of cruelty.[60]

What *** is suggesting here echoes Bayle's discussion of the virtuous atheist in the *Pensées diverses sur la comète* [Diverse Thoughts on the Comet] (1st ed. 1682), as well as his appearance in some articles of Bayle's *Dictionaire historique et critique* [Historical and Critical Dictionary] (1697), notably 'Spinoza' and 'Epicurus'. Both the content and the elliptical style recall Bayle, who presented the idea of a virtuous atheist as a kind of paradox. Indeed of Epicurus, Bayle says, 'on ne saurait dire assez de bien de l'honnêteté de ses mœurs, ni assez de mal de ses opinions sur la religion. Une infinité de gens sont orthodoxes et vivent mal; lui, au contraire, et plusieurs de ses sectateurs avaient une mauvaise doctrine et vivaient bien' [not enough good can be said about the honesty of his morals and not enough bad about his opinions of religion. An infinite number of people are orthodox and live badly; he, by contrast, and many of his followers had a bad doctrine but lived well].[61] We have already seen that Saunderson expresses Epicurean views, and his virtue now provokes the same observations that Epicurus' did. Saunderson thus seems to be what Bayle calls 'un athée de naissance' [an atheist from birth or, more appropriately here, a man-born-atheist], morally superior to those who positively decide to be atheists and who give atheists in general a

59 DPV, 4, p. 52; Hobson and Harvey, p. 63; *Letter*, pp. 202–3.
60 DPV, 4, p. 51; Hobson and Harvey, p. 62; *Letter*, p. 201.
61 Bayle, *Dictionnaire*, vol. 2, p. 370.

bad name. Bayle says, 'Or, parce que ceux qui étouffent ou qui tâchent d'étouffer dans leur âme par belle malice la connaissance de Dieu sont les plus insignes débauchés et les plus déterminés pêcheurs qui soient au monde, on se persuade que tous les athées indifféremment sont des scélérats' [So because those who, out of superb malice, suffocate or try to suffocate the knowledge of God in their souls are the most signal of libertines and determined of sinners that there have ever been, we convince ourselves that any and every atheist is a villain].[62]

The paradox of Sanderson's blind yet moral life and of his seeing the light at the end, despite being blind, is given a further twist as ***'s commentary on his last words continues, and he expands the set of metaphors of the senses to include hearing and the lack of it. He declares, 'La voix de la nature se fait entendre suffisamment à lui à travers les organes qui lui restent, et son témoignage n'en sera que plus fort contre ceux qui se ferment opiniâtrement les oreilles et les yeux' [The voice of nature can make itself heard clearly enough through his remaining organs and his testimony will thereby be an even greater challenge to those who stubbornly shut their eyes and ears].[63] Saunderson was merely blind and not deaf, and so while he could not see nature's marvels, he could hear them. However, the reference to another sense organ merely displaces the problem of belief: a voice may guarantee the blind can be faithful and/or virtuous, but it leaves men-born-blind-and-deaf naturally atheist.[64] Metaphors of revelation shortly reappear, however, though they are now accompanied by a reference to a Socrates that has an unsettling effect. *** says, 'Je demanderais volontiers si le vrai Dieu n'était pas encore mieux voilé pour Socrate par les ténèbres du paganisme, que pour Saunderson par la privation de la vue et du spectacle de la nature' [I should willingly ask whether the true God was not more veiled to Socrates by the pagan darkness than he was to Saunderson, whose blindness deprived him of the spectacle of nature].[65] At one level, the hypothetical question suggests that in a Christian era, there is no excuse for atheism since even a blind man can see the light, but at another level, if the question is hypothetical, perhaps it is because the reference to Socrates introduces an example of

62 Pierre Bayle, *Pensées sur la comète*, A. Prat (ed.), 2 volumes (Paris: Droz, 1939), vol. 2, pp. 121–2.

63 DPV, 4, p. 53; Hobson and Harvey, p. 63; *Letter*, p. 203.

64 A reference to 'the voice of nature' can be found in, for example, the Port-Royal edition of Pascal's *Pensées* (1670), which speaks of atheists as deaf to 'cette voix de la nature qui a retenti continuellement à leurs oreilles' [this voice of nature that has continually resounded in their ears]. (*Pensées de M. Pascal sur la Religion et sur quelques autres sujets*, édition de Port-Royal (1670) et ses compléments (1678–1776), Georges Couton and Jean Jehasse (eds) (Saint Etienne: Editions de l'Université, 1971), p. 263).

65 DPV, 4, p. 53; Hobson and Harvey, p. 63; *Letter*, p. 203.

a virtuous pagan which lends further support to the possibility that the Christian faith is not a necessary condition for virtuous life.[66]

And as if to confirm Saunderson in the image of the virtuous atheist, *** reports a second account of his death. It is probably also supposed to be taken from Inchlif, though its relationship to the one reported previously is deliberately unclear: where does it belong in the fictional chronology, or is it an alternative to the conversation with Holmes? He is shown dying surrounded by his family in a sentimental scene:

> Les derniers adieux qu'il fit à sa famille sont fort touchants. 'Je vais', leur dit-il, 'où nous irons tous; épargnez-moi des plaintes qui m'attendrissent. Les témoignages de douleur que vous me donnez, me rendent plus sensible à ceux qui m'échappent. Je renonce sans peine à une vie qui n'a été pour moi qu'un long désir, et qu'une privation continuelle. Vivez aussi vertueux et plus heureux; et apprenez à mourir aussi tranquilles'. Il prit ensuite la main de sa femme, qu'il tint un moment serrée entre les siennes: il se tourna le visage de son côté, comme s'il eût cherché à la voir; il bénit ses enfants, les embrassa tous, et les pria de se retirer, parce qu'ils portaient à son âme des atteintes plus cruelles que les approches de la mort.[67]

> His final farewell to his family is very touching: 'I am going,' he told them, 'where we all go. Spare me your distress, which I feel moved by. The signs of pain that escape your lips only make me more sensitive to the ones that elude my grasp. I feel no sorrow at leaving a life that has been nothing more to me than one long deprivation and endless yearning. Live as virtuously as I have and more happily, and learn to die as peacefully.' With that he took his wife's hand and held it tight in his for a while. Then he turned to face her as though he were trying to see her, blessed his children, embraced them all and begged them to withdraw as their presence was a crueller pain for his soul than the approach of death.[68]

The contrast with his loquaciousness in Holmes's presence is remarkable. There is perhaps a slight sense of the pastiche about this sentimental scene as the dying virtuous blind man mimes the gestures of the dying sighted,

66 For a study of the uses to which the figure of Socrates is put in early modern writing, see Jean-Pierre Cavaillé, 'Socrate libertin' in *Socrate in Occidente*, Ettore Lojacono (ed.) (Grassina: Le Monnier, 2004), pp. 33–65.

67 DPV, 4, p. 53–4; Hobson and Harvey, p. 64.

68 *Letter*, p. 203.

turning to face his wife whom he cannot see.[69] Yet the comparison with the recognition scenes of the cataract narratives, with which we began and in which tears of joy were shed, also brings Saunderson's words about his life being 'one long deprivation and endless yearning' into sharper focus. Not only do they contrast with the man-born-blind-of-Puiseaux's cheeky sense of his blind superiority, but they also will echo in ***'s discussion of Molyneux's Problem, to which Madame is – finally – going to get a solution, and in which blindness as pain and suffering, physical and metaphysical, is an unexpectedly important theme.

69 For a different reading of the scene, see Caroline Warman, 'Intimate, Deprived, Uncivilised: Diderot and the Publication of the Private Moment', in Andrew Kahn (ed.), *Representing Privates Lives of the Enlightenment*. *SVEC*, 2010: 11, 35–51.

Six

Dis/Solving Molyneux's Problem

So the time has come for an explicit examination of Molyneux's Problem, as *** declares, 'On cherche à restituer la vue à des aveugles-nés' [People are trying to give sight to those born blind].[1] Of course, by this point in the *Letter*, the context for an examination of the Problem has changed, and ***'s use of the third-person impersonal pronoun 'on' [people] suggests he is continuing to distance himself from attempts to make the blind see. We recall *** saying in the opening paragraph of the *Letter* that he had never thought anything would be learnt from the experiment done by one person in particular, Réaumur, but that he had originally thought the problem would lie with either Madame or Mademoiselle Simoneau. We still don't know why. Before revealing the answer and turning to the examination of Molyneux's Problem, to the way in which *** subtly revises some of his earlier claims regarding the relationship between touch and sight, and to the theological considerations to which this gives rise, we must consider what the operation itself entailed and who it was that Réaumur had invited to perform it, namely the Prussian oculist, Joseph Hillmer.

The Prussian's Girl-Born-Blind

Like the English oculist, Grant, to whom we referred in the Prologue, Hillmer was a travelling oculist.[2] A sense of his services can be gained from this flyer, available in Leipzig in 1746:

> Der 24sten September. Frühe um 10 Uhr ist honetten Personen erlaubt zuzuschauen, wie er stockblinde sehend macht, mehrentheils mit seinem geheimen Augen-Geist in einer Minuten; solcher dienet sehr wohl allen blöden Gesichtern; Dergleichen geheime Medecinische Kleinodien er mehr besitzet in hinfallender Sucht, Schwindsucht, Venus-Krankheiten, Fieber, Haupt. Magen, und Weiber-Zuständ, auch taube und lahme damit zu curieren.

1 DPV, 4, p. 54; Hobson and Harvey, p. 65; *Letter*, p. 204.

2 See Aloys Henning, *Die Affäre Hillmer: Ein Okulist aus Berlin in Petersburg 1751* (Frankfurt: Peter Lang, 1987).

> NB. Die Armen mögen sich nur gleich bey Zeiten melden um mit Proben umsonst an ihnen zu zeigen.[3]
>
> On the 24th September at 10 in the morning, good people are invited to witness him give sight to the blind using his secret eye-potion that works in minutes. It also works on other eye problems. He has other precious medical secrets for use in cases of fainting, consumption, venereal disease, fever, headaches, stomach-aches and women's pains. The deaf and lame can also be cured by them.
>
> NB. The poor may come along at the stated time to volunteer to be tested on free of charge.

Hillmer's quackery is self-evident to us today, though it did not strike everyone at the time: in 1748. Frederick the Great conferred on Hillmer the title of court eye surgeon and, thus elevated, Hillmer set off for Paris where Réaumur seems to have been impressed too. Others in Paris seem to have thought his skills rather more dubious, however: on 21 August 1749, Condillac wrote to the Swiss mathematician, Gabriel Cramer, telling him that the Prussian oculist was off to Geneva, having acquired 'une réputation assez équivoque' [a rather uncertain reputation] in Paris. Strangely, he recommends him nonetheless to Cramer, perhaps making a joke about the clear-sighted vision of the Protestant Genevans: '[j]'apprends qu'il va à Genève. Je compte qu'il y sera mieux jugé qu'ailleurs. Si vous avez quelque aveugle né, je vous le recommande' [I discover he is going to Geneva. I expect him to be judged more favourably there than elsewhere. If you have a blind man, I recommend him to you].[4] By the early 1750s, however, Hillmer's reputation was over. As Aloys Hennings has shown in *Die Affäre Hillmer* (1987), he would be expelled from St Petersburg for charlatanism.

Did Diderot know or suspect that Hillmer's operating skills were never such that they were likely to afford any light to either patients or spectators? *** refers to Hillmer as 'le Prussien' [the Prussian],[5] a term that might conceivably be derogatory, but there are no other clues. What *** is interested in is the nature of the operation and, in particular, the pain involved in it and the delicate nature of the eye. We will remain with Hillmer for a little longer to explore this.

---

3 Henning, *Die Affäre Hillmer*, pp. 62–3.

4 Condillac, *Lettres inédites à Gabriel Cramer* (Paris: Presses Universitaires de France, 1953), p. 54. I am grateful to Wes Williams for the suggestion that the reference to Geneva might be read this way.

5 DPV, 4, p. 29: Hobson and Harvey, p. 39; *Letter*, p. 181.

A Painful Operation

Nineteenth-century medical historians have a tendency to present early modern surgeons as butchers. However, even if we account for a degree of macabre exaggeration, there can be little doubt that Hillmer's operations were not without some serious discomfort for his patients. The following account of one of Hillmer's operations is taken from a nineteenth-century German history of eye surgery:

> He inserted a round, fairly blunt needle through the vitreous humour to the back of the lens which he then detached at the top and went round the edge of it with the needle so quickly that it fell into the vitreous humour along with the cataract. Then he inserted the needle into the lens again and pulled it back into the opening he had made, where it was then to graft itself in place and never slide up again. In the case of a soft and milky cataract, he would go round the lense with the needle five or six times. After the operation, Hillmer was satisfied if the patient could see a box or a clock, and paid no more attention to him, leaving it to his assistant, who would later become an oculist himself, to bandage the patient's eye. He took some of his master's volatile eye potion in his hands and let it evaporate in the patient's eye. Then they applied whisked egg-white mixed with crushed alum and camphor which the assistants charged the patient an extra *thaler*. Hillmer operated with such impertinent audacity and was so rough that when one woman shrieked in pain, he gave her a clip round the ear, when he already had his needle in her eye. After the bandaging was done, the patient could go home, either by carriage or by horse or on foot. A few days later, almost all of them were inoperably blind. Hillmer did not wait to find out. He took his money and disappeared. Of the fifty people he operated on in the Lübeck region, only four retained their sight.[6]

Certainly nothing could be further removed from the painless, instantaneous transformation imagined in Molyneux's Problem or reported in either *Tatler* or the Gospels.

The *Letter* refers explicitly to the operation as 'douloureuse' [painful].[7] Moreover, it raises the question as to whether the sense of sight is worth the pain or not. Though it sounds as though Saunderson might have wished to see, since he experienced his blindness as deprivation, the man-born-blind of Puiseaux had, we recall, no desire to see and said he would much rather have longer arms than the sense of sight. The possibility

6 Quoted in German in Henning, *Die Affäre Hillmer*, p. 61.
7 DPV, 4, p. 54; Hobson and Harvey, p. 65; *Letter*, p. 204.

of a blind man not wishing to see might be said to bring into focus Molyneux's phrase about the man-born-blind being '*made* to see' (my emphasis). Molyneux meant nothing coercive by his phrasing, of course; his Problem is non-surgical, a thought-experiment, but it would not stay that way. Voltaire says of the boy-born-blind that Cheselden persuaded him to have the operation, but that 'il eut de la peine à y consentir' [he had difficulty consenting to it].[8] We are not told of the events leading up to Mademoiselle Simoneau's operation. Perhaps she did wish for sight, but we might wonder whether the earlier references to compassion and the blind's lack of it might not be extended to Réaumur, whose vanity was so blinding that he had Hillmer perform an operation, of which the pain was certain and the success of its outcome far from assured.

If sight is not acquired painlessly and its merits not universally acclaimed, it is not acquired instantaneously either. *** describes the physiology of the eye at length, suggesting that after the painful operation, the patient should not instantly be exposed to light and would wish to sit in varying degrees of darkness while recovering. Certainly the last thing s/he would want straight after cataract surgery is to be asked to solve an epistemological brainteaser such as Molyneux's: 'je ne conçois pas, je l'avoue, ce que l'on espère d'un homme à qui l'on vient de faire une opération douloureuse, sur un organe très délicat que le plus léger accident dérange et qui trompe souvent ceux en qui il est sain et qui jouissent depuis longtemps de ses avantages' [I cannot, I confess, understand what it is hoped might be gained from a man who has just undergone a painful operation on a very sensitive organ which is disturbed by the slightest accident and often deceives those in whom it is healthy and who have enjoyed its benefits for some time].[9] So, assuming Hillmer was able to make Simoneau's daughter see and that she consented to this, the question remains as to whether she would be able to answer the question in Molyneux's Problem. What did *** mean when he said he had thought that she would be at fault in Réaumur's experiment not being instructive?

Trained Eyes

Before he examines Molyneux's question and the existing answers, *** asserts that the question is much more difficult than it might seem. It would certainly be beyond the grasp of Mademoiselle Simoneau and beyond that of Madame too or, at least, it would have been before she had read the *Letter*. The subject would need not only to be able to see but also to be able to reflect on what it was they were seeing, and the same is true of the witnesses who would need, in addition, to be able to understand

8 Voltaire, *Œuvres complètes*, vol. 15, p. 319.
9 DPV, 4, p. 54; Hobson and Harvey, p. 65; *Letter*, p. 204.

the answer they heard the subject give. That is to say, they would all need to be philosophers, which neither Mademoiselle Simoneau nor Madame is because, as women and, in the case of the former, possibly of the artisan class, they have not received sufficient education. *** observes, '[s]i l'on voulait donner quelque certitude à des expériences, il faudrait du moins que le sujet fût préparé de longue main, qu'on l'élevât, et peut-être qu'on le rendît philosophe' [if the experiments were to be at all reliable, the subject would need, at least, to have been be prepared for them a long time in advance, and have been brought up as and perhaps made into a philosopher].[10] Moreover, becoming or, rather, being made into a philosopher 'n'est pas l'ouvrage d'un moment' [cannot be done overnight].[11] It is not enough simply to open your eyes and see; accessing truth is not, we understand, like faith.

Nothing could be further removed from Foucault's account of the mythical foundation of Enlightenment philosophy, which was, we recall, the 'bright, distant, open naïvety of the gaze'. The gaze envisaged by *** is, by contrast, far from naïve, indeed he envisages no less than the combined talents of Newton, Descartes, Locke and Leibniz as suitable instructors for the man-born-blind. As for witnesses to the event, *** says the experiment should take place in an entirely academic context or, rather, he says, again maliciously if implicitly sniping at Réaumur and implying that membership of the Academy is not necessarily the mark of a suitable spectator, that only those with appropriate levels of philosophical and anatomical knowledge should be invited to witness the event. This would exclude Madame.

This reference to the reliability of subjects and witnesses has implications for the biblical stories and, moreover, it recalls the discussion of miracles in Diderot's earlier work, the *Pensées philosophiques*. While Pascal's *Pensées* challenged the reader to believe what he saw or to believe what he read in the Bible about what others saw, in spite of the fact that it went against his reason, many of the *Pensées philosophiques* claim, *pace* Pascal, that seeing and reading are not believing. The thinker of 'Pensée L' [Thought 50] triumphantly declares:

> Grâce à l'extrême confiance que j'ai en ma raison, ma foi n'est point à la merci du premier saltimbanque. Pontife de Mahomet, redresse des boiteux; fais parler des muets; rends la vue aux aveugles; guéris des paralytiques; ressuscite des morts; restitue même aux estropiés les membres qui leur manquent, miracle qu'on n'a point encore tenté: et à ton grand étonnement ma foi ne sera point ébranlée. Veux-tu que

10 DPV, 4, p. 55; Hobson and Harvey, p. 65; *Letter*, p. 204.
11 DPV, 4, p. 55; Hobson and Harvey, p. 65; *Letter*, p. 204.

> je devienne ton proselyte? Laisse tous ces prestiges, et raisonnons. Je suis plus sûr de mon jugement que de mes yeux.[12]
>
> Thanks to the great confidence I have in my reason, my faith is not at the mercy of every charlatan. Mohammed the Pontiff, cure cripples, make mutes speak and blind men see, cure the lame, bring the dead back to life, even restore missing limbs to the maimed, a miracle that has not yet been tried, and to your great astonishment, my faith will not waver. Do you want me to become your follower? Then forget all these tricks, and let's reason. I am more certain of my judgement than my eyes.

This dogmatic tone is far stronger than that of *** in the *Letter* – only Saunderson's speech comes close to it. However, the requirement in the *Letter* that the subject and the witnesses of the experiment designed to determine the answer to Molyneux's question should be philosophers is borne of the same view. As *** puts it:

> J'aurais moins de confiance dans les réponses d'une personne qui voit pour la première fois, que dans les découvertes d'un philosophe qui aurait bien médité son sujet dans l'obscurité; ou, pour vous parler le langage des poètes, qui se serait crevé les yeux pour connaître plus aisément comment se fait la vision.[13]
>
> I should have less confidence in the responses of a man seeing for the first time than in the discoveries of a philosopher who had meditated long and hard on the matter in the dark or, to put it in poetic terms, had gouged out his eyes, the more comfortably to discover the workings of vision.[14]

We find here an echo of the earlier reference to 'a man who had only been able to see for a day or two' and whose reports of visual phenomena were believed by the blind and disbelieved by the freethinkers. There are other links to the *Pensées philosophiques* too: 'Pensée LIII' notes the role of rumour in the fabrication of miracle narratives, which points to the hearsay on which *** said Réaumur hoped to rely for the enhancement of his reputation.[15]

If Réaumur is not named again here, he is certainly alluded to. The pomposity of the Academician and his blindness to his inability to provide

12 DPV, 2, p. 45.
13 DPV, 4, p. 54–5; Hobson and Harvey, p. 65.
14 *Letter*, p. 204.
15 DPV, 2, p. 47.

Mademoiselle Simoneau with the right sort of philosophical preparation is suggested here in the comic use of the impersonal pronoun 'on' [one]: 'ce n'est pas l'ouvrage d'un moment, que de faire un philosophe, même quand on l'est; que sera-ce, quand on ne l'est pas? C'est bien pis quand on croit l'être' [making someone a philosopher cannot be done overnight, even when one is a philosopher onself; and how long would it take if one were not? It takes even longer when one thinks one is].[16] So what exactly is at stake in the question that needs a philosopher to answer it and philosophers to hear the answer?

Seeing the Light

The matter is complex. What was at stake in the question differed from one philosopher's speculative response to the next and, moreover, the empirical data provided by the English surgeon, Cheselden, and his boy patient from Newington Butts, altered the stakes further. In the *Letter*, having examined the first question as to whether the ideas of cubes and spheres could be obtained from touch at all (and answered in the affirmative), and having established that the patient would be unlikely to be able to see anything much immediately after the operation, *** observes that Molyneux's question in fact comprises a number of different questions that require separate examination. These are whether the subject would in due course be able visually to distinguish shapes, whether s/he would recognize them as the same shapes as s/he had touched earlier, and whether it would be possible to provide a demonstration that this was indeed the case. As we'll see, in ***'s discussion, the relations between touch and sight that were suggested in some of the earlier discussion are reversed, and Saunderson's suffering is given a significant role.

*** devotes a great deal of space to the first of these questions which arises in response to Condillac, who was in turn responding to Voltaire. In the *Eléments de la philosophie de Newton* (1738), Voltaire had reported Cheselden's observations and concluded that he had proved both Locke and Berkeley right when they asserted that it was only by combining the experience of sight and touch that it was possible to see shapes.[17] Yet Berkeley had gone further than Locke and argued that touch alone could procure the subject ideas of size and shape, a position also held earlier by ***. Condillac challenged Voltaire's reading of Cheselden's data: referring to his own experience, he says that when he sees cubes and spheres, he is not aware of combining a haptic idea with the visual one, and so there is no reason to suppose that the man-born-blind-and-made-to-see would do so either. To Condillac, if Cheselden's experiment appeared to suggest the

---

16 DPV, 4, p. 55; Hobson and Harvey, p. 65; *Letter*, p. 204.

17 Voltaire, *Eléments de la philosophie de Newton mis à la portée de tout le monde*, in *Œuvres complètes*, vol. 15, p. 319.

boy needed touch to be able to see, it was simply because his eyes were insufficiently recovered from the operation.[18]

*** now agrees with Condillac's critique of Berkeley's view of the primacy of touch; indeed, he is most insistent that the eye functions independently of the hand:

> Pour s'assurer par le toucher, de l'existence et de la figure des objets, il n'est pas nécessaire de voir; pourquoi faudrait-il toucher pour s'assurer des mêmes choses par la vue? Je connais tous les avantages du tact, et je ne les ai pas déguisés, quand il a été question de Saunderson ou de l'aveugle du Puiseaux; mais je ne lui ai point reconnu celui-là.[19]

> In order to be sure of the existence and shape of the objects we touch, we do not need to be able to see them. Why then would we need to touch objects in order to be sure we could see them? I am aware of all the benefits of touch, and I did not disguise them when I was discussing Saunderson or the blind man of Puiseaux; that, however, was not one I recognized.[20]

He repeats this view later, providing a number of examples in which the hand is more easily deceived than the eye. He tells Madame, for example, that if a very thin piece of paper had been placed between her fingers, she would only know it was there if she saw it.[21] With respect to the earlier comparison between how the sighted and a man-born-blind think, *** seems to have changed his mind: touch is no longer necessary for the idea of shape.

Before we observe the implications for the other two questions that form Molyneux's Problem, we must consider what the implications of this change of position might be. Is the *Letter* beginning to restore sight to its former glory?

Metaphysical Pain

It seems to be hard to praise sight or even simply make the case for its independence from touch without some kind of theological interference. Diderot no doubt knew that Condillac had ended his defence of the eye's

18 Etienne Bonnot de Condillac, *Essai sur les connaissances humaines*, in *Œuvres philosophiques*, Georges Le Roy (ed.), 3 volumes (Paris: Presses Universitaires de France, 1947), vol. 1, pp. 58–9; *Essay on the Origin of Human Knowledge*, Hans Aarsleff (trans.) (Cambridge: Cambridge University Press, 2001), p. 108–9.

19 DPV, 4, p. 62; Hobson and Harvey, p. 72.

20 *Letter*, pp. 210–11.

21 DPV, 4, pp. 62–3; Hobson and Harvey, p. 72; *Letter*, p. 211.

ability to see shapes without the aid of touch as follows:

> Il serait curieux de découvrir les lois que Dieu suit, quand il nous enrichit des différentes sensations de la vue; sensations qui non seulement nous avertissent mieux que toutes les autres des rapports des choses à nos besoins et à la conservation de notre être, mais qui annoncent encore, d'une manière bien plus éclatante, l'ordre, la beauté et la grandeur de l'univers.[22]

> It would be interesting to discover the laws that God follows when He enriches us with the different sensations of sight, sensations that not only inform us better than all the others about how things relate to our needs and preservation, but that also in a much more striking way proclaim the order, beauty and grandeur of the universe.[23]

*** does not quote this part of the *Essai* in the *Letter*, but central to his discussion of Molyneux's question is Saunderson's view of blindness, which is not that of the man-born-blind of Puiseaux; for Saunderson, blindness is misfortune and loss. *** observes:

> Encore une fois, que peut-on attendre de précis de celui qui n'a aucune habitude de réfléchir et de revenir sur lui-même, et qui, comme l'aveugle de Cheselden, ignore les avantages de la vue, au point d'être insensible à sa disgrâce, et de ne point imaginer que la perte de ce sens nuise beaucoup à ses plaisirs? Saunderson à qui l'on ne refusera pas le titre de philosophe, n'avait certainement pas la même indifference.[24]

> I say it again, how precise can one expect someone to be, if they are not used to thinking and self-examination, and if they, like Cheselden's blind man, are so unaware of the benefits of sight that they are unaware of their misfortune and cannot imagine how the loss of this sense impairs their pleasures? Saunderson, whom we cannot refuse the title of philosopher, was certainly not indifferent to his loss.[25]

The man-born-blind of Puiseaux and Saunderson may both be blind, but the former's nonchalant attitude to his blindness is itself a lack, and one for which he is here unfavourably compared to Saunderson.

---

22 Condillac, *Œuvres*, vol. 1, p. 57.
23 Condillac, *Essay*, p. 106.
24 DPV, 4, p. 65; Hobson and Harvey, pp. 75–6.
25 *Letter*, p. 213.

The comparison contests what Voltaire had called a 'vérité importante' [important truth], namely the Montaignian view that 'il est impossible d'être malheureux par la privation des biens dont on n'a pas d'idée' [it is impossible to be unhappy as a result of being deprived of things one has no idea of], which he said was demonstrated by the fact that Cheselden's boy had no desire to see.[26] By contrast, Saunderson is shown here to have an idea of what he lacks and, moreover, as he told his family, he experiences his deprivation as very painful – not physically (as its restoration might be), but metaphysically.

Having just agreed with Condillac's *Essai*, *** now disputes a point in the *Traité des systèmes*, in which Condillac gives an account of the origin of the idea of the gods. It derives, he says, as indeed all rational thought for Condillac, from changes in our perception that permit comparison, which is the most basic form of thought. He says (and *** quotes):

> si la vie de l'homme n'avait été qu'une sensation non interrompue de plaisir ou de douleur, heureux dans un cas sans aucune idée de malheur, malheureux dans l'autre sans aucune idée de bonheur, il eût joui ou souffert; et que, comme si telle eût été sa nature, il n'eût point regardé autour de lui, pour découvrir, si quelque être veillait à sa conservation, ou travaillait à lui nuire.[27]

> if man's life had been nothing other an uninterrupted sensation of pleasure or pain, either happy with no idea of unhappiness, or unhappy with no idea of happiness, he would have known only pleasure or suffering; and, as if that were his very nature, he would never have looked around to see whether some being was keeping a protective watch over him or plotting to do him harm.[28]

For Condillac, this primitive idea of a being that seeks to harm or protect, acquired on the basis of changes in the nature of our perceptions, is to be contrasted with the true idea of God, which civilized man subsequently acquires. For polemical purposes, however, *** presents it as his account of the sensationist origin of the idea of God, and he disputes it.

It is not so much the idea of such a being that he disputes, nor does he dispute that the idea of his existence is dependent on the experience of pain or pleasure; instead he rejects the claim that a man whose only experience was painful would be unable to acquire the idea of his existence. Pain, he argues, is not like light and dark that can only be known

26 Voltaire, *Œuvres complètes*, vol. 15, p. 319.
27 Condillac, *Traité des systèmes*, in *Œuvres philosophiques*, vol. 1, p. 134; DPV, 4, p. 65–6; Hobson and Harvey, p. 76.
28 *Letter*, pp. 213–14.

in relation to each other. Suffering is absolute, not relative – indeed it seems to be the only thing in the *Letter* that isn't. And so while it might be true, he says, that a man whose only experience was painful might not know the difference between his sensation and his existence underlying it, nothing would stop him from crying out, 'Qu'ai-je fait, pour exister?' [What have I done to exist?].[29] And because suffering does not relate to pleasure as darkness does to light, *** can draw on what Saunderson said about his life to suggest that to be born blind is to suffer, that a man-born-blind is a man-born-in-pain. This involves a shift in the grounds for theological discussion with respect to the earlier part of the *Letter*: whereas the man-born-blind had no access to (what the sighted claimed was) the visible, marvellous evidence for God's existence, he does have the evidence of his own physical suffering, which prompts him to pose the metaphysical and ontological question, 'What have I done to exist?'.

With regard to physical suffering, *** explains further, '[i]l eût été très naturel de le regarder comme un état forcé, de se sentir innocent, de se croire pourtant coupable et d'accuser ou d'excuser la nature, tout comme on fait' [it would have been perfectly natural to think of it as an enforced condition, to feel oneself innocent, yet believe oneself to be guilty, and blame or excuse nature, which is what we do].[30] There are some important moves here: the shift in tense (from conditional past to indicative), which itself enables the shift in value of the third-person impersonal pronoun (from 'it' and 'one' to 'we'), turns Condillac's hypothetical man-born-in-pain into a real person, perhaps the man-born-blind, and that real person into a figure for all humanity. The man-born-blind is thus no longer the exceptional figure he was earlier: his suffering makes him the same as everyone else and, moreover, it is this common experience that produces the idea of God.

The idea is not, however, without an internal contradiction and a mystery as *** observes that we feel innocent but our suffering makes us believe we are guilty, of what we do not know. We might expect a reference and a challenge to the doctrine of original sin here. Indeed, in the unpublished *De la Suffisance de la Religion Naturelle* [On the Sufficiency of Natural Religion] (1746), Diderot had described that doctrine, as Saunderson had described Holmes's God, that is, in terms of elephants and tortoises,[31] but here *** says no more, and man's suffering remains an inexplicable or, at least, unexplained fact of his life.

Of course, such theological speculation leaves Molyneux's question

---

29 DPV, 4, p. 66; Hobson and Harvey, p. 76; *Letter*, p. 214.
30 DPV, 4, p. 66; Hobson and Harvey, p. 76; *Letter*, p. 214.
31 DPV, 2, p. 192.

still unanswered. Now, finally (should we still care about it), *** gives us his answer to Molyneux's question or, rather, his answers.

It Depends

If you were to ask Mademoiselle Simoneau whether she could tell that the shapes she could see were the same shapes as the ones she had touched, she would not understand the implications of the question and would simply guess the answer. Her testimony would therefore provide no secure foundation for knowledge. A reliable answer could be obtained, *** explains, from either a metaphysician or a mathematician, or, rather, each would provide a reliable but different answer.

Had Locke been born blind and the experiment been done on him, he would have had a full understanding of the question and its implications, but he would quickly have begun to doubt: he would have wondered whether, even if he could believe what others told him – namely that things that can be seen can also be touched (which is, of course, not the case for the mirror image, which cannot be touched) – he could not have been sure that the same object did not feel different to the hand to the way it appeared to the eye. Locke's answer would be, *** says, 'Messieurs [. . .] ce corps me semble le carré, celui-ci le cercle; mais je n'ai aucune science qu'ils soient tels au toucher qu'à la vue' [Gentlemen [. . .] this body seems to me to be the square and this the circle, but I cannot know for certain that they feel the same as they look].[32] His answer might be reliable, but it involves the claim that he has no reliable knowledge.

Had Saunderson been made to see, however, he would have fared rather better. This is because circles and squares are amenable to geometrical demonstration. *** imagines he would have said:

> Ceux à qui je démontrais les propriétés du cercle et du carré, n'avaient pas les mains sur mon abaque, et ne touchaient pas les fils que j'avais tendus et qui limitaient mes figures; cependant ils me comprenaient. [. . .] Ainsi voilà ce que j'ai toujours nommé carré, et voilà ce que j'ai toujours nommé cercle.[33]

> Those people who witnessed my demonstration of the properties of the circle and the square did not have their hands on my abacus, and they couldn't touch the threads I had tied to make the outlines of my shapes; yet they could understand me. [. . .] So that's what I have always called a square, and that's what I have always called a circle.[34]

---

32 DPV, 4, p. 68; Hobson and Harvey, p. 78; *Letter*, p. 216.
33 DPV, 4, p. 69; Hobson and Harvey, p. 79.
34 *Letter*, p. 216.

As Colas Duflo has observed, the suggestion here is not that a geometer's ability to answer correctly proves that the mind is furnished with some kind of innate geometrical ideas, for *** envisages Saunderson performing a geometrical demonstration to other people. Geometry is understood here as a human convention rather than as some kind of eternal truth.[35] Moreover, as *** is quick to point out, most human experience does not involve cubes and spheres, and had Saunderson been asked to identify any other object, he would have failed. Geometry might solve Molyneux's Problem, but social customs and habits pose much greater problems to a man-born-blind-and-made-to-see. It is with respect to these customs that what Foucault described as the naïve eye now makes another appearance.

Saunderson would assume that the shape of an object, which he has been trained to recognize by way of properties, went, as it were, hand in hand with its function. As a result, though he might be able to recognize that his skullcap is something he wears on his head, the function of his mortarboard with its square shape and purely decorative tassle would remain a mystery to him. However, his inability to work it out would provide material for an excellent satire on 'ce que nous appellons le bon goût' [what we call good taste].[36] Yet no sooner has the naïve eye been shown to see through custom than it is shown to make mistakes: Saunderson would also take a man sitting still for a piece of furniture or a machine, and a tree swaying in the wind for 'un être se mouvant, animé et pensant' [a self-moving, animate and thinking being].[37] While such errors appear to cast the thinking matter hypothesis, discussed earlier, as an elementary error that a more experienced eye will correct, the example of the tree might also be read as a satirical reference to the Gospel of St. Mark, in which the man Jesus made to see initially thought men were 'trees, walking'.[38] Moreover, it is followed by an observation that recalls the earlier reference to thinking matter as a hypothesis based on the experience of touch: 'Madame, combien nos sens nous suggèrent de choses; et que nous aurions de peine sans nos yeux, à supposer qu'un bloc de marbre ne pense ni ne sent!' [Madame, how many things our senses suggest to us, and if we didn't have eyes, how difficult we would find it to suppose that a block of marble could not think and feel!].[39] The suggestion is that touch constantly makes the same mistake as the inexperienced eye: whereas with experience, the sighted are able to see that marble can't see, whenever the blind feel marble, they feel it touching them and thus assume it is sensate too. *** presents such a claim as absurd, but given the frequently ironic status

35 Duflo, *Diderot philosophe*, p. 149.
36 DPV, 4, p. 70; Hobson and Harvey, p. 80; *Letter*, p. 217.
37 DPV, 4, p. 70; Hobson and Harvey, p. 80; *Letter*, p. 218.
38 Mark 8: 24.
39 DPV, 4, p. 70; Hobson and Harvey, p. 80; *Letter*, p. 218.

of his exclamatory register, it is also suggested that what the naïve eye sees and what the hand feels is a truth to which experience has made the sighted blind. If Saunderson's newly sighted eye provides material for a satire on 'good taste', perhaps it also reveals the belief in dualism to be a mere custom of mind.

In a final twist, however, the knowledge we gain from our senses, be they visual or haptic, experienced or not, is reduced by ***, in a manner that recalls Saunderson's 'single dot', to 'presque rien' [almost nothing]. He claims that our senses tell us nothing about the nature of matter, thought, movement, space and time, and that even true mathematical definitions are, like one of the shapes they define, circular. He says, 'quand on a mis les connaissances humaines dans la balance de Montaigne, on n'est pas éloigné de prendre sa devise [. . .] Nous ne savons donc presque rien' [once we have weighed human knowledge in Montaigne's scales, we are not far from adopting his motto [. . .] We know therefore almost nothing].[40]

Of course, as many readers have noted, 'not being far from' adopting something is not the same as actually adopting it, and the claim is that we know 'almost nothing' rather than nothing at all. However, as we'll see by way of conclusion, what *** focuses on in his final lines is not so much to do with what we do or do not know as it is to do with the means by which we go about knowing anything: conversation.

40 DPV, 4, p. 72; Hobson and Harvey, p. 82; *Letter*, p. 219.

Conclusion, or Two Hours Later . . .

*** signs off as follows:

> Nous ne savons donc presque rien: cependant combien d'écrits dont les auteurs ont tous prétendu savoir quelque chose. Je ne devine pas pourquoi le monde ne s'ennuie point de lire, et de ne rien apprendre, à moins que ce ne soit par la même raison qu'il y a deux heures que j'ai l'honneur de vous entretenir, sans m'ennuyer et sans vous rien dire. Je suis avec un très profond respect,
>
> MADAME,
>
> votre très humble et très obéissant serviteur.
>
> *** [1]

> We know therefore almost nothing, and yet how many works there are whose authors have all claimed to know something. I cannot imagine why people do not tire of reading and yet learning nothing, unless it is for the same reason that I have had the honour of conversing with you for two hours without either boring myself or saying anything to you. I am, with the deepest respect,
>
> MADAME,
>
> your most humble and most obedient servant.
>
> *** [2]

His concluding *captatio benevolentiæ* puts the emphasis not so much on knowledge as on the pleasures of conversation. It was all about talking, not about saying anything. His letter has privileged blind, phatic communication over the referent-laden kind because it was less boring, more fun.

This ending is not simply to be dismissed as ironic as it has so often been by readers who take the *Letter* to contain a clear statement of

1 DPV, 4, p. 72; Hobson and Harvey, p. 82.
2 *Letter*, p. 219.

Diderot's atheist materialism. I think we should take it seriously because the text has indeed been fun to read, precisely because *** kept saying almost nothing to the reader, either because he was reporting what other people said or because he either couldn't say the half of what he knew or couldn't know the half of what he said. And as a participant in this game of nods and winks, nudges and whispers, the reader has been enjoying supplying half the ideas and half the words for herself. She has taken her place in the enlivening and enlightening conversation that is the *Letter*.

Some of the moments when the reader was required to come up with the ideas or the words were, we recall, signalled visually – typographically – and it is to typography that *** once again has recourse to ensure his very final message is conveyed. His deepest respect for the reader is made visible in the capitalisation of 'MADAME', and his self-effacing modesty is shown by the reduction of the font size for his signature. And it is here that blindness and enlightenment can finally and clearly be seen together: in the paradoxical inky glimmer of three little stars.

Bibliography

Primary sources

Anonymous, *Dissertation sur la formation du monde (1738); Dissertation sur la résurrection de la chair (1743): manuscrits du recueil 1168 de la Bibliothèque Mazarine de Paris,* Stancati, Claudia (ed.) (Paris: Champion, 2001).

Anonymous, *Lazarillo de Tormes and The Swindler: Two Spanish Picaresque Novels,* Alpert, Michael (trans., intro. and notes) (London: Penguin, 2003).

Anonymous, *Le garçon et l'aveugle: jeu du XIIIe siècle,* Dufournet, Jean (trans., ed. and comm.) (Paris: Champion, 2007).

Balzac, Jean Louis Guez, seigneur de, *Œuvres,* Moreau L., (ed.), 2 volumes (Paris: J. Lecoffre, 1854).

Bayle, Pierre, *Dictionnaire historique et critique,* fifth edition, 4 volumes (Amsterdam, Leiden, The Hague, Utrecht, 1740).

——, *Pensées sur la comète,* Prat, A. (ed.), 2 volumes (Paris: Droz, 1939).

——, *Œuvres diverses,* Labrousse, Elisabeth (ed.), 9 volumes (Hildesheim: G. Olms, 1964–90).

de Bergerac, Cyrano, *L'Autre monde: ou, Les états et empire de la lune* in *Œuvres complètes,* Madeleine Alcover (ed.), 3 volumes (Paris: Champion, 2000), vol. 1.

——, *Œuvres complètes,* Alcover, Madeleine (ed.), 3 volumes (Paris: Champion, 2000).

——, *Journey to the Moon,* Brown, Andrew (trans.) (London: Hesperus, 2007).

Berkeley, George, *New Theory of Vision,* second edition (Dublin: Printed by Aaron Rhames for Jeremy Pepyat, 1709).

——, *Three Dialogues between Hylas and Philonous* (London: printed by G. James for Henry Clements, 1713).

——, *The Analyst; or, A Discourse addressed to an infidel Mathematician: Wherein it is examined whether the Object, Principles, and Inferences of the modern Analysis are more distinctly conceived, or more evidently deduced, than religious Mysteries and Points of Faith* (London: Printed for J. Tonson in the Strand, 1734).

——, *A Defence of Free-Thinking in Mathematics in answer to a Pamphlet of Philalethes Cantabrigiensis, intituled, Geometry no Friend to Infidelity, or a Defence of Sir Isaac Newton, and the British Mathematicians* (London: Printed for J. Tonson in the Strand, 1735).

——, *Dialogues entre Hylas et Philonous* (Amsterdam, 1744).

——, *The Works of George Berkeley, Bishop of Cloyne*, Luce, A. A. and Jessop, T. E. (eds), 9 volumes (London: Nelson, 1948–64).

——, *A Treatise Concerning the Principles of Human Knowledge*, Dancy, Jonathan (ed.) (Oxford: Oxford University Press, 1998).

Boullier, David Renaud, 'Lettre de M. Gervaise Holmes à l'auteur de la *Lettre sur les aveugles*, contenant le véritable récit des dernières heures de Saounderson, à Cambridge, MDCCL', *Journal des savants* (Amsterdam edition) March 1752, 516–44.

——, 'Observations au sujet d'un Ecrit intitulé: Lettre sur les aveugles, à l'usage de ceux qui voient. Londres, MDCCXLIX', *Journal des savants* (Amsterdam edition) May 1752, 471–521.

Brantôme, Pierre de Bourdeille, Seigneur de, *Discours sur les colonels de l'infanterie de France*, Vaucheret, Etienne (ed.), with a preface by V. -L. Saulnier (Paris: Vrin, 1973).

Buffon, Georges Leclerc, comte de, *Histoire naturelle, générale et particulière, avec la description du cabinet du roy*, 36 volumes (Paris: Imprimerie royale, 1749–88).

Clément, Pierre, 'Lettre XXXIII' (20 June 1749), in *Les Cinq années littéraires ou Lettres de M. Clément sur les ouvrages de littérature qui ont paru dans les années 1748, 1749, 1750, 1751 et 1752*, 4 volumes (Berlin: Sous le bon plaisir des souscripteurs et se distribuent chez les Libraries les plus consciencieux et les plus désintéressées, 1754), vol. 1, pp. 185–6.

Charron, Pierre, *Toutes les Œuvres de Pierre Charron, Parisien, Docteur es Droicts, Chantre et Chanoine Theologal de Condom. Dernière edition. Reveuës, corrigées & augmentées*, 2 volumes (Paris: Jacques Villery, 1635).

Cheselden, William, 'An Account of some Observations Made by a Young Gentleman, Who Was Born Blind, or Lost His Sight so Early, That He Had no Remembrance of Ever Having Seen, and Was Couch'd Between 13 and 14 Years of Age'. *Philosophical Transactions of the Royal Society*, vol. 35 (1727–1728) (London: W. Innys, 1665–1886), pp. 447–50.

Condillac, Etienne Bonnot de, *Œuvres philosophiques*, Le Roy, Georges (ed.), 3 volumes (Paris Presses Universitaires de France, 1947).

——, *Essay on the Origin of Human Knowledge*, Hans Aarsleff (trans.), (Cambridge: Cambridge University Press, 2001).

——, *Lettres inédites à Gabriel Cramer*, texte établi, présenté et annoté par Georges Le Roy (Paris: Presses Universitaires de France, 1953).

Descartes, René, *Discours de la méthode* (Paris: Nicolas Poisson, 1724).

——, *Œuvres de Descartes*, Adam, Charles and Tannery, Paul (eds), 11 volumes (Paris: Vrin, 1964–76).

——, *The Philosophical Writings of Descartes*, Cottingham, John, Stoothoff, Robert and Murdoch, Dugald (trans.), 3 volumes (Cambridge: Cambridge University Press, 1985).

Diderot, Denis, *Lettre sur les aveugles*, Niklaus, Robert (ed.) (Geneva: Droz, 1951).

——, *Correspondance*, Roth, Georges and Varloot, Jean (eds), 16 volumes (Paris: Minuit, 1955–70).

——, *Œuvres philosophiques*, Vernière, Paul (ed.) (Paris: Garnier, 1956).

——, *Œuvres complètes*, Herbert Dieckmann, Jacques Proust and Jean Varloot (eds), 30+ volumes (Paris: Hermann, 1975–).

——, *Œuvres*, Versini, Laurent (ed.), 5 volumes (Paris: Robert Laffont, 1994–97).

——, *Lettre sur les aveugles. Lettre sur les sourds et muets*, Hobson, Marian and Harvey, Simon (eds) (Paris: Garnier-Flammarion, 2000).

Diderot, Denis, and d'Alembert, Jean, *Encyclopédie, ou Dictionnaire raisonné des sciences, des arts et des métiers*, 28 volumes (Paris: Le Breton, Briasson, David and Durand, 1751–72).

du Fouilloux, Jacques, *La Vénerie* (Poitiers, 1561).

Dyer, George, *The Privileges of the University of Cambridge*, 2 volumes (London: Longman, 1824).

Empiricus, Sextus, *Outlines of Scepticism*, Julia Annas and Jonathan Barnes (ed. and trans.) (Cambridge: Cambridge University Press, 2000), pp. 26–7.

Estienne, Charles, *Paradoxes*, Peach, Trevor (ed.) (Geneva: Droz, 1998).

Fontenelle, Bernard Le Bovier de, *Entretiens sur la pluralité des mondes* (Amsterdam: Chez Pierre Mortier, 1687).

Formey, Henri-Samuel, *Lettre de M. Gervaise Holmes à l'auteur de la Lettre sur les aveugles, contenant le véritable récit des dernières heures de Saounderson* (Cambridge, 1750).

——, 'Remarques sur l'Article concernant la *Lettre de M. Gervaise Holmes*, qui a été inséré dans le *Journal des Savants*, edit. d'Amst. Mars 1752, p. 516 et suiv', in *Bibliothèque impartiale*, May–June 1752, 443–6.

Gassendi, Pierre, *Disquisitio metaphysica; seu, Dubitationes et instantiae adversus Renati Cartesii Metaphysicam et responsa. Recherches métaphysiques; ou, Doutes et instances contre la Métaphysique de R. Descartes et ses réponses*, Rochot, Bernard (ed.) (Paris: Vrin, 1962).

Graffigny, Françoise de, *Lettres d'une Péruvienne*, Mallinson, Jonathan (ed.) (Oxford: Voltaire Foundation, 2002).

Hobbes, Thomas, *The English Works of Thomas Hobbes, now first collected and edited by Sir William Molesworth*, 11 volumes (London: J. Bohn, 1839–45).

Hume, David, *An Enquiry concerning Human Understanding*, Millican, Peter (ed.) (Oxford: Oxford University Press, 2007).

La Chapelle, Jean-Baptiste de, *Institutions de géométrie*, third edition, 2 volumes (Paris: chez Debure l'Aîné, 1757).

La Mettrie, Julien Offray de, *Histoire naturelle de l'âme traduite de l'anglois de M. Charp, par M. H** de l'Académie des sciences. Nouvelle édition revue fort exactement, corrigée de quantité de fautes & augmentée de la lettre critique de M. de la Mettrie à Madame la marquise du Châtelet* (Oxford [Paris]: Aux dépends de l'auteur, 1747).

——, *L'Homme Machine: A Study in the Origins of an Idea*, Vartanian, Aram (ed.) (Princeton: Princeton University Press, 1960).
——, *Machine Man and other writings*, Thomson, Ann (ed.) (Cambridge: Cambridge University Press, 1996).
La Mothe Le Vayer, François de, *Œuvres*, 7 volumes (Dresden: Michel Groell, 1756).
Le Blanc, Jean-Bernard, *Lettres d'un Français*, 2 volumes (The Hague: Jean Neaulme, 1745).
Le Grand, Marc-Antoine, *L'aveugle clairvoyant* in M. Claude-Bernard Petitot, *Répertoire du théâtre français*, 23 volumes (Paris: Didot l'aîné, 1803–4), vol. 18, pp. 356–406.
Lelarge de Lignac, Joseph Adrien, *Lettres à un Américain sur l'histoire naturelle, générale et particulière de Monsieur de Buffon*, 5 volumes (Hamburg: n.p., 1751).
The Leibniz-Clarke Correspondence, Alexander, H. G. (ed.) (Manchester: Manchester University Press, 1956).
Locke, John, *The Correspondence of John Locke*, de Beer, E. S. (ed.), 9 volumes (Oxford: Clarendon Press, 1976–89).
——, *An Essay Concerning Human Understanding*, Nidditch, Peter H. (ed. and foreword) (Oxford: Oxford University Press, 1979).
Lucretius, *On the Nature of the Universe*, Melville, Ronald (trans.), Fowler, Don and Peta (intro. and notes) (Oxford World's Classics, 1997).
Maillet, Benoît de, *Telliamed, ou, entretiens d'un philosophe indien avec un missionnaire français sur la diminution de la mer, nouv. éd. rev. cor. et aug. sur les originaux de l'auteur, avec une vie de M. de Maillet* (La Haye: Chez Duchesne, 1755).
Mandeville, Bernard, *By a Society of Ladies: Essays in The Female Tatler*, Goldsmith, M. M. (ed.) (Bristol: Thoemmes, 1999).
Marana, Giovanni Paolo, *L'Espion turc dans les cours des princes chrétiens, ou lettres et mémoires d'un envoyé secret de la Porte dans les cours de l'Europe*, 7 volumes (Londres: Aux dépens de la Compagnie, 1742).
Marivaux, Pierre Carlet de Chamblain de, *Le Cabinet du philosophe* (Paris: Prault, 1734).
Meslier, Jean, *Œuvres complètes*, Deprun, Jean, Desné, Roland, Soboul, Albert (eds), 3 volumes (Paris: Editions Anthropos, 1970–72).
Molière, *Œuvres complètes*, Forestier, Georges (ed.), 2 volumes (Paris: Gallimard, 2010).
Montaigne, Michel de, *Essais*, Villey-Saulner (ed.), (Paris: Presses Universitaires de France, 2004).
——, *The Complete Works: Essays, Travel Journal, Letters*, Frame, Donald M. (trans.), Hampshire, Stuart (intro.) (London: Everyman, 2003).
Newton, Isaac, *Méthode des fluxions et des suites infinies* (Paris: chez de Bure l'aîné, 1740).
Paré, Ambroise, *Les Œuvres d'Ambroise Paré, conseiller et premier chirurgien du roy, divisées en vingt-sept livres: avec les figures et portraicts tant de*

l'Anatomie que des instruments de chirurgie et de plusieurs monstres: reveuz et augmentez par l'autheur pour la seconde édition (Paris: Gabriel Buon, 1579).

Pascal, Blaise, *Œuvres complètes*, Lafuma, Louis (ed.) (Paris: Editions du Seuil, 1963).

——, *Pensées de M. Pascal sur la Religion et sur quelques autres sujets*, édition de Port-Royal (1670) et ses compléments (1678–1776), Couton, Georges and Jehasse, Jean (eds) (Saint Etienne: Editions de l'Université, 1971).

——, *Pensées and Other Writings*, Levi, Honor (trans.), Levi, Anthony (intro. and notes) (Oxford: Oxford World's Classics, 2008).

Piles, Roger de, *Cours de peinture par principes* (Paris: Jombert, 1766).

Polignac, Melchior de, *Anti-Lucretius, sive De Deo et natura, libri novem* (Paris: Henri-Louis Guerin and Jean Guerin, 1747).

Raphson, Joseph, *Analysis æquationum universalis, seu, Ad æquationes algebraicas resolvendas methodus generalis, & expedita, ex nova infinitarum serierum methodo, deducta ac demonstrata. Editio secunda cum appendice; cui annexum est, De spatio reali, seu entre infinito conamen mathematico-metaphysicum* (London: Typis T. Braddyll, prostant venales apud Johannem Taylor, 1697).

Réaumur, René Antoine Ferchault, seigneur de, *Mémoires pour servir à l'histoire des insectes*, 6 volumes (Paris: Imprimerie Royale, 1734–42).

Rougeart, Jucquel, *Œuvres completes (1578)*, Magnien-Simonin, Catherine (ed.) (Geneva: Droz, 1988).

Rousseau, Jean-Jacques, *Œuvres complètes*, Gagnebin, Bernard and Raymond, Marcel (eds), 5 volumes (Paris: Gallimard, 1959–97).

——, *Confessions*, Scholar, Angela (trans.), Coleman, Patrick (ed., intro. and notes) (Oxford: Oxford World's Classics, 2008).

Saunderson, Nicholas, *The Elements of Algebra, in Ten Books: by Nicholas Saunderson LL.D. Late Lucasian Professor of the Mathematics in the University of Cambridge, and Fellow of the Royal Society. To which is prefixed, an account of the author's life and character, collected from his oldest and most intimate acquaintance*, 2 volumes (Cambridge, Printed at the University-Press, and sold by Mrs. Saunderson at Cambridge, by John Whiston bookseller at Boyle's Head in Fleet Street London, and Thomas Hammond in York, 1740).

Sextus Empiricus, *Outlines of Scepticism*, Annas, Julia and Barnes, Jonathan (trans. and ed.) (Cambridge: Cambridge University Press, 2000).

Shaftesbury, Anthony Ashley Cooper, Third Earl of, *Characteristics of Men, Manners, Opinions, Times*, Klein, Lawrence E. (ed.) (Cambridge: Cambridge University Press, 1999).

The Spectator, Bond, Donald F. (ed.), 5 volumes (Oxford: Clarendon Press, 1965).

Tallement, Gédéon, sieur des Réaux, *Historiettes*, Adam, Antoine (ed.), 2 volumes (Paris: Gallimard, 1960–61).

The Tatler, Bond, Donald F. (ed.), 3 volumes (Oxford: Clarendon Press, 1987).

Toland, John, *Letters to Serena* (London: Printed for Bernard Lintot, 1704).

Voltaire, *Œuvres complètes* (Oxford: Voltaire Foundation, 1968–).

Secondary Sources

Adams, D. J., *Diderot, Dialogue and Debate* (Liverpool: Cairns, 1986).
Anderson, Wilda, *Diderot's Dream* (Baltimore: Johns Hopkins University Press, 1990).
Ballstadt, Kurt, *Diderot: Natural Philosopher*. *SVEC*, 2008: 09.
Barach, Moshe, *Blindness: The History of a Mental Image in Western Thought* (New York: Routledge, 2001).
Beauchet-Filleau, H. (ed.), *Dictionnaire historique et généalogique des familles du Poitou* (Poitiers: Oudin, 1891–1979).
Bennett, Jonathan, 'Substratum'. *History of Philosophy Quarterly*, 4.2 (1987), 197–215.
Berchielli, Laura, 'Colour, Space and Figure in Locke: An Interpretation of the Molyneux Problem'. *Journal of the History of Philosophy*, 40.1 (2002), 47–65.
Bloch, Olivier, *Le matérialisme au siècle des Lumières* (Paris: Presses Universitaires de France, 1992).
Bonnefon, Paul, 'Diderot à Vincennes'. *Revue de l'Histoire Littéraire de la France*, 6 (1899), 200–24.
Bourdin, Jean-Claude, *Diderot. Le matérialisme* (Paris: Presses Universitaires de France, 1998).
——, 'Matérialisme et scepticisme chez Diderot'. *Recherches sur Diderot et l'Encyclopédie*, 26 (1999), 85–97.
——, 'Le matérialisme dans la *Lettre sur les aveugles*'. *Recherches sur Diderot et l'Encyclopédie*, 28 (2000), 83–96.
Bracken, H. M., *The Early Reception of Berkeley's Immaterialism, 1710–1733* (The Hague: Nijhoff, 1959).
Brennan, Teresa, and Jay, Martin, *Vision in Context: Historical and Contemporary Perspectives on Sight* (London: Routledge, 1996).
Brewer, Daniel, *The Discourse of Enlightenment in Eighteenth-Century France: Diderot and the Art of Philosophizing* (Cambridge: Cambridge University Press, 1993).
Cabane, Franck, *L'écriture en marge dans l'œuvre de Diderot* (Paris: Champion, 2009).
Cantor, Geoffrey, 'Berkeley's *The Analyst* revisited', *Isis*, 75.4 (1984), 668–83.
Cavaillé, Jean-Pierre, *Descartes. La fable du monde* (Paris: Vrin, 1991).
——, *Dissimulations. Religion, morale et politique au XVIIe siècle* (Paris: Champion, 2002).
——, 'Socrate libertin', in Lojacono, Ettore (ed.), *Socrate in Occidente* (Grassina: Le Monnier, 2004), 33–65.
Cave, Terence, *Pré-histoires. Textes troublés au seuil de la modernité* (Geneva: Droz, 1999).
——, *Retrospectives: Essays in Literature, Poetics and Cultural History*, Kenny, Neil and Williams, Wes (eds) (Oxford: Legenda, 2009).
Chabut, Marie-Hélène, 'La *Lettre sur les aveugles*: l'écriture comme écart'. *SVEC*, 304 (1992), 1245–9.

Charles, Sébastien, *Berkeley au siècle des lumières: immatérialisme et scepticisme au XVIIIe siècle*, with a preface by Geneviève Brykman (Paris: Vrin, 2003).
——, 'De Popkin à Rousseau: retour sur le scepticisme des Lumières'. *Philosophiques*, 35.1 (2008), 275–90.
Charrak, André, 'Géométrie et métaphysique dans la *Lettre sur les aveugles* de Diderot'. *Recherches sur Diderot et l'Encyclopédie*, 28 (2000), 43–53.
Chartier, Roger, *Les origines culturelles de la révolution française* (Paris: Seuil 1990).
——, *The Cultural Origins of the French Revolution*, Cochrane, Lydia G. (trans.) (Durham, NC: Duke University Press, 1991).
Chottin, Marion (ed.), *L'aveugle et le philosophe* (Paris: Presses Universitaires de Paris-Sorbonne, 2009).
Chouillet, Anne-Marie, 'Trois lettres inédites de Diderot'. *Recherches sur Diderot et l'Encyclopédie*, 11 (1991), 10–17.
Chouillet, Jacques, *La formation des idées esthétiques de Diderot* (Paris: Armand Colin, 1973).
Clark, Stuart, *Vanities of the Eye: Vision in Early Modern European Culture* (Oxford: Oxford University Press, 2007).
Colie, Rosalie Littell, *Paradoxa Epidemica: The Renaissance Tradition of Paradox* (Princeton: Princeton University Press, 1966).
Copenhaver, Brian T., 'Jewish Theologies of Space in the Scientific Revolution: Henry More, Joseph Raphson, Isaac Newton and their Predecessors'. *Annals of Science*, 37.5 (1980), 489–548.
Cronk, Nicholas, 'Voltaire and the Benefits of Censorship: The Example of the *Lettres philosophiques*', in Johnson, E. Joe and Wells, Byron R. (eds), *An American Voltaire: Essays in Memory of J. Patrick Lee* (Newcastle Upon Tyne: Cambridge Scholars Publishing, 2009), 33–61.
Curran, Andrew, *Sublime Disorder: Physical Monstrosity in Diderot's Universe*. *SVEC*, 2001: 1.
Daniel, Georges, *Le style de Diderot: légende et structure* (Paris and Geneva: Droz, 1986).
Daniel, Stephen H., 'Berkeley's Pantheistic Discourse'. *International Journal for Philosophy of Religion*, 49 (2001), 179–94.
Darnton, Robert, *The Business of Enlightenment: a Publishing History of the Encyclopédie, 1775–1800* (Cambridge, MA: Bellknap Publishing, 1979).
——, 'Les Encyclopédistes et la police', *Recherches sur Diderot et l'Encyclopédie*, 1 (1986), 94–109.
Daston, Lorraine and Park, Katherine, *Wonders and the Order of Nature, 1150–1750* (Cambridge, MA: Zone Books, 1998).
Dear, Peter, 'The Meanings of Experience', in Lindberg, David C. and Numbers, Ronald L. (eds), *The Cambridge History of Science*, 7 volumes (Cambridge: Cambridge University Press, 2003), vol. 3, 106–31.
Derrida, Jacques, *De la grammatologie* (Paris: Minuit, 1967).
——, *Of Grammatology*, Spivak, Gayatri (trans.) (Baltimore: Johns Hopkins University Press, 1976).
——, *Mémoires d'aveugle: l'autoportrait et autres ruines* (Paris: Réunion des Musées Nationaux, 1991).

——, *Memoirs of the Blind: The Self-Portrait and other Ruins*, Pascale-Anne Brault and Michael Naas (trans.) (Chicago: University of Chicago Press, 1993).

Duflo, Colas, *Diderot philosophe* (Paris, Champion, 2003).

Evans, G. R., 'The Molyneux Question', in *Gareth Evans: Collected Papers* (Oxford: Clarendon Press, 1985), 364–99

Farrell, Gabriel, *The Story of Blindness* (Cambridge Mass.: Harvard University Press, 1956).

Feldherr, Andrew, 'Ships of State: *Aeneid* 5 and Augustan Circus Spectacle'. *Classical Antiquity*, 14.2 (1995), 245–65.

Floridi, Luciano, *Sextus Empiricus: The Transmission and Recovery of Pyrrhonism* (Oxford: Oxford University Press, 2002).

Fontenay, Elisabeth de, *Diderot ou le matérialisme enchanté* (Paris: Grasset, 1981).

Foucault, Michael, *Naissance de la clinique* (Paris: Presses Universitaires de France, 1963).

——, *The Birth of the Clinic*, Sheridan, A. M. (trans.) (London: Tavistock, 1973).

Gaukroger, Stephen, '"Home Alone": Cognitive Solipsism in the Early-Modern Era'. *Proceedings and Addresses of the American Philosophical Association*, 80.2 (2006), 63–78.

Giocanti, Silvia, 'La Mothe Le Vayer: modes de diversion sceptique'. *Libertinage et philosophie au XVIIe siècle*, 2 (1997), 33–48.

Guicciardini, Niccolò, 'Newton's method and Leibniz's calculus', in Jahnke, Hans Niels (ed.), *A History of Analysis* (The American Mathematical Society, 2003), 73–104.

Glauser, Richard, 'Diderot et le problème de Molyneux'. *Etudes philosophiques* (1999), 291–327.

Goodden, Angelica, *Diderot and the Body* (Oxford: Legenda, 2001).

Groult, Martine, 'La question de Molyneux et la notion d'expérience. Une entente parfaite entre Diderot et d'Alembert'. ~~*VOIR*~~, 19 (1999), 52–67.

Hall, A. Rupert, *Philosophers at War: the Quarrel between Newton and Leibniz* (Cambridge: Cambridge University Press, 1980).

Hankins, Thomas L., *Science and the Enlightenment* (Cambridge: Cambridge University Press, 1985).

Hanks, Lesley, *Buffon avant l'histoire naturelle* (Paris: Presses Universitaires de France, 1966).

Hartmann, Pierre, *Diderot. La figuration du philosophe* (Paris: José Corti, 2003).

Hayhoe, Simon, *God, Money, and Politics: English Attitudes to Blindness and Touch, from the Enlightenment to Integration* (Charlotte: Information Age Publishing, 2008).

Hellegouarc'h, Jacqueline, 'Les aveugles juges de couleurs: interprétation et essai de datation'. *SVEC*, 215 (1982), 91–7.

Heller-Roazen, Daniel, *The Inner Touch: Archeology of a Sensation* (Cambridge: MIT Press, 2007).

Hellerstedt, Kahren Jones, 'The Blind Man and his Guide'. *Netherlands Quarterly for the History of Art*, 13.3/4 (1983), 163–81.

Henning, Aloys, *Die Affäre Hillmer: Ein Okulist aus Berlin in Petersburg 1751* (Frankfurt am Main: Peter Lang, 1987).
——, 'Diderot, the European Underground and English Radical Thought: Filling in the Gaps', in *Diderot and European Culture*, Ogée, Frédéric and Strugnell, Anthony (eds), *SVEC*, 2006: 09, 145–57.
——, *Diderot and Rousseau: Networks of Enlightenment. Collected Essays by Marian Hobson*, Tunstall, Kate E. and Warman, Caroline (trans. and intro), *SVEC*, 2011: 4.
Hobson, Marian, *The Object of Art: Theories of Illusion in Eighteenth-Century France* (Cambridge: Cambridge University Press, 1982, repr. 2009).
Israel, Jonathan, *Radical Enlightenment: Philosophy and the Making of Modernity, 1650–1750* (Oxford: Oxford University Press, 2001).
Jacob, Margaret C., *Radical Enlightenment: Pantheists, Freemasons and Republicans* (London and Boston: George Allen and Unwin, 1981).
Jacot Grapa, Caroline, *Dans le vif du sujet: Diderot, corps et âme* (Paris: Classiques Garnier, 2009).
Jay, Martin, *Downcast Eyes: The Denigration of Vision in Twentieth-Century French Thought* (Berkeley: University of California Press, 1994).
Jesseph, Douglas M., 'Leibniz on the Foundations of the Calculus: The Question of the Reality of Infinitesimal Magnitudes'. *Perspectives on Science*, 6.1–2 (1998), 6–40.
Kafker, Frank A., 'The Recruitment of the Encyclopedists'. *Eighteenth-Century Studies*, 6.4 (Summer, 1973), 452–61.
Kafker, Frank A. and Loveland, Jeff, 'The Elusive Laurent Durand, a Leading Publisher of the French Enlightenment'. *SVEC*, 12: 2005, 223–58.
——, 'Diderot et Laurent Durand, son éditeur principal.' *Recherches sur Diderot et l'Encyclopédie*, 39 (2005), 29–40.
Kaitaro, Timo, *Diderot's Holism* (Frankfurt am Main: Peter Lang, 1997).
Kelly, Mary Byrd, 'Saying by Implicature: The Two Voices of Diderot in *La Lettre sur les aveugles*'. *Studies in Eighteenth-Century Culture*, 12 (1983), 231–41.
Kessler, Michael, 'A Puzzle Concerning Diderot's Presentation of Saunderson's "Palpable Arithmetic"'. *Diderot Studies*, 20 (1981), 159–7.
Klein, Lawrence, 'Enlightenment as Conversation', in Baker, Keith, and Reill, Peter (eds), *What's Left of Enlightenment? A Postmodern Question* (Stanford: Stanford University Press, 2001), 148–66.
Knox, Kevin C., *From Newton to Hawking: a History of Cambridge University's Lucasian Professors of Mathematics* (Cambridge: Cambridge University Press, 2003).
Krakeur, Lester Gilbert and Krueger, Raymond Leslie, 'The Mathematical Writings of Diderot', *Isis*, 33: 2 (June 1941), 219–32.
Koyré, Alexander, *From the Closed World to the Infinite Universe* (New York: Harper, 1958).
Larrissy, Edward, *The Blind and Blindness in Literature of the Romantic Period* (Edinburgh: Edinburgh University Press, 2007).

Le Ru, Véronique, 'La *Lettre sur les aveugles* et le bâton de la raison'. *Recherches sur Diderot et l'Encyclopédie*, 28 (2000), 25–41.
Levin, Janet, 'Molyneux's Question and the Individuation of Perceptual Concepts'. *Philosophical Studies*, 139 (2008), 1–28.
Lichtenstein, Jacqueline, *La couleur éloquente: rhétorique et peinture à l'âge classique* (Paris: Flammarion, 1989).
——, *The Eloquence of Colour: Rhetoric and Painting in the French Classical Age*, McVarish, Emily (trans.) (Berkeley: University of California Press, 1993).
——, *La tache aveugle: essai sur les relations de la peinture et de la sculpture à l'âge moderne* (Paris: Gallimard, 2003).
——, *The Blind Spot: An Essay on the Relations Between Painting and Sculpture in the Modern Age*, Miller, Chris (trans.) (Los Angeles: Getty Publications, 2008).
Lojkine, Stéphane, 'Beauté aveugle et monstruosité sensible: le détournement de la question esthétique chez Diderot (la *Lettre sur les aveugles*)', in Cottegnies, Line, Gheeraert, Tony and Venet, Gisèle (eds), *La beauté et ses monstres dans l'Europe baroque* (Paris: Presses de la Sorbonne Nouvelle, 2003), 61–78.
Lough, John, *Essays on the Encyclopédie of Diderot and D'Alembert* (London: Oxford University Press, 1968).
Maia Neto, José R., and Popkin, Richard H., (eds), *Skepticism in Renaissance and Post-Renaissance Thought: New Interpretations* (New York: Humanity Books, 2004).
Maurseth, Anne Beate, *L'analogie et le probable: Pensée et écriture chez Denis Diderot*. *SVEC*, 2007: 09.
Mandelbrote, Scott, 'Newton and Eighteenth-Century Christianity', in Cohen, I. Bernard and Smith, George E. (eds), *The Cambridge Companion to Newton* (Cambridge: Cambridge University Press, 2002), 409–30.
Markovits, Francine, 'Mérian, Diderot et l'aveugle', in J. -B. Mérian, *Sur le problème de Molyneux*, with a postface by Francine Markovitz (Paris: Flammarion, 1984), 193–282.
——, 'L'aveugle, une figure de la philosophie sceptique', ~~*VOIR*~~, 19 (1999), 34–51.
McLean, Ian (ed.), *Heterodoxy in Early Modern Science and Theology* (Oxford: Oxford University Press, 2001).
Mehlman, Jeffrey, *Cataract, a Study in Diderot* (Middletown, CN: Wesleyan University Press, 1979).
Milam, Jennifer, 'Fragonard and the Blindman's Game'. *Art History*, 21.1 (1998), 1–25.
Moreau, Isabelle, *'Guérir du sot': les stratégies d'écriture des libertins à l'âge classique* (Paris: Champion, 2007).
Moriarty, Michael, *Early Modern French Thought: The Age of Suspicion* (Oxford: Oxford University Press, 2003)
——, *Fallen Nature, Fallen Selves: Early Modern French Thought II* (Oxford: Oxford University Press, 2006).
Morin, Robert, *Diderot et l'imagination* (Paris: Les Belles Lettres, 1987).

——, *Les Pensées philosophiques de Diderot devant leurs principaux contradicteurs au XVIIIe siècle* (Paris: Les Belles Lettres, 1975).

Nakagawa, Hisayasu, 'Diderot, Rousseau et autres "incrédules" au service du catholicisme: à propos du *Déisme réfuté par lui-même* de l'abbé Bergier'. *Recherches sur Diderot et l'Encyclopédie*, 39 (2005), 157–76.

Ogée, Frédéric, and Strugnell, Anthony (eds), *Diderot and European Culture. SVEC*, 2006: 09.

O'Gorman, Ellen, *Irony and Misreading in the Annals of Tacitus* (Cambridge: Cambridge University Press, 2000).

Pasini, Enrico, 'Arcanum Artis Inveniendi: Leibniz and Analysis', in Otte, Michael, and Panza, Marco (eds), *Analysis and Synthesis in Mathematics: History and Philosophy* (Dordrecht: Kluwer, 1997), 35–46.

Paterson, Mark, *The Senses of Touch: Haptics, Affects and Technologies* (Oxford: Berg, 2007).

Paulson, William R., *Enlightenment, Romanticism and the Blind in France* (Princeton: Princeton University Press, 1987).

Pedersen, John, 'La complicité du lecteur dans l'œuvre de Diderot: à propos de la *Lettre sur les aveugles*', *Actes du 6ème Congrès des Romanistes Scandinaves* (Stockholm: Almqvist & Wiksell, 1977), 205–10.

Petitot, M. Claude-Bernard, *Répertoire du théâtre français*, 23 volumes (Paris: Didot l'aîné, 1803–4).

Pintard, René, *Le libertinage érudit dans la première moitié du XVIIe siècle*, 2 volumes (Paris: Boivin, 1943).

Pommier, Jean, *Diderot avant Vincennes* (Paris: Boivin et cie, 1939).

Popkin, Richard H., *The History of Scepticism: From Savonarola to Bayle* (Oxford: Oxford University Press, 2003).

Prigogine, Ilya, and Stengers, Isabelle, *Order Out of Chaos: Man's New Dialogue with Nature* (London: Heinemann, 1984).

——, *La nouvelle alliance: métamorphose de la science* (Paris: Gallimard, 1986).

Proust, Jacques, 'L'Initiation artistique de Diderot'. *Gazette des Beaux-Arts*, 55 (1960), 225–32.

——, *Diderot et l'Encyclopédie* (Paris: Albin Michel, 1962).

Pycior, Helena M., *Symbols, Impossible Numbers and Geometric Entanglements* (Cambridge: Cambridge University Press, 1997).

Quintili, Paolo, *La pensée critique de Diderot: matérialisme, science et poésie à l'âge de l'Encyclopédie (1742–1782)* (Paris: Champion, 2001).

——, *Matérialismes et lumières: philosophies de la vie, autour de Diderot et de quelques autres, 1706–1789* (Paris: Champion, 2009).

Rex, Walter E., *Diderot's Counterpoints: the Dynamics of Contrariety in his Major Works. SVEC*, 1998: 363.

Riskin, Jessica, *Science in the Age of Sensibility* (Chicago: University of Chicago Press, 2002).

Roger, Jacques, *Les sciences de la vie au XVIIIe siècle* (Paris: A. Colin, 1963).

——, *The Life Sciences in Eighteenth-Century French Thought*, Benson, Keith R. (ed.), Ellrich, Robert (trans.) (Stanford: Stanford University Press, 1993).

Roger, Jacques, 'Diderot et Buffon en 1749' *Diderot Studies*, 4 (1962), 221–36.
Sacks, Oliver, *The Man Who Mistook his Wife for a Hat* (New York: Summitt Books, 1985).
——, *An Anthropologist on Mars* (New York: Vintage, 1995).
Salaün, Franck, *L'ordre des mœurs: essai sur la place du matérialisme dans la société française du XVIIIe siècle (1734–1784)* (Paris: Editions Kimé, 1996).
——, (ed.), *Diderot–Rousseau: un entretien à distance* (Paris: Desjonquères, 2006).
Sassen, Brigitte, 'Kant on Molyneux's Problem'. *British Journal for the History of Philosophy*, 12.3 (2004), 471–85.
Scholar, Richard, *The Je-Ne-Sais-Quoi in Early Modern Europe: Encounters with a Certain Something* (Oxford: Oxford University Press, 2005).
——, *Montaigne and the Art of Free-Thinking* (Oxford: Peter Lang, 2011).
Schwartz, Jerome, *Diderot and Montaigne. The Essais and the Shaping of Diderot's Humanism*, (Geneva: Droz, 1966).
Shea, Louise, *The Cynic Enlightenment: Diogenes in the Salon* (Baltimore: Johns Hopkins University Press, 2010).
Singh, Christine M., 'The *Lettre sur les aveugles*: Its Debt to Lucretius', *Studies in Eighteenth-Century French Literature* (Exeter, University of Exeter, 1975), 233–42.
Spary, Emma, *Utopia's Garden: French Natural History from Old Regime to Revolution* (Chicago: Chicago University Press, 2000).
Starobinski, Jean, 'Sur l'emploi du chiasme dans *Le Neveu de Rameau*'. *Revue de métaphysique et de morale*, 89.2 (1984), 182–96.
Steczowicz, Agnieszka, *The Defence of Contraries: Paradox in the Late Renaissance Disciplines* (Oxford D. Phil, 2004).
Steintrager, James A., *Cruel Delight: Enlightenment Culture and the Inhuman* (Bloomington: Indiana University Press, 2004).
Stenger, Gerhardt, 'La théorie de la connaissance dans la *Lettre sur les aveugles*'. *Recherches sur Diderot et l'Encyclopédie*, 26 (1999), 99–111.
Strugnell, Anthony, 'La candidature de Diderot à la Société Royale de Londres'. *Recherches sur Diderot et l'Encyclopédie*, 6 (1989), 37–41.
Strugnell, Anthony, 'Diderot chercheur: du nouveau sur les emprunts faits par Diderot à la Bibliothèque royale entre 1775 et 1782'. *Recherches sur Diderot et l'Encyclopédie*, 8 (1990), 12–19.
Teyssèdre, Bernard, *Roger de Piles et les débats sur le coloris au siècle de Louis XIV* (Paris: Bibliothèque des Arts, 1964).
Thomson, Ann, *Bodies of Thought: Science, Religion, and the Soul in the Early Enlightenment* (Oxford: Oxford University Press, 2008).
Torlais, Jean, *Réaumur: un esprit encyclopédique en dehors de l'Encyclopédie* (Paris: Librairie Blanchard, 1961).
Trousson, Raymond, *Diderot jour après jour: chronologie* (Paris: Champion, 2006).
Tunstall, Kate E., '"Des circonstances assez peu philosophiques": Diderot's 'aveugle-né du Puiseaux', *French Studies Bulletin*, 99 (2006), 33–6.
——, 'Paradoxe sur le portrait: auto-portrait de Diderot en Montaigne'. *Diderot Studies*, 30 (2007), 197–210.

——, 'The Judgement of Experience: Reading and Seeing in Diderot's *Lettre sur les aveugles*'. *French Studies*, 62.4 (2008), 404–16.

——, 'L'Aveugle qui suit l'aveugle qui suit l'aveugle: la philosophie intertextuelle de la *Lettre sur les aveugles*', in Chottin, Marion (ed.), *L'Aveugle et le philosophe*, (Paris: Presses Universitaires de Paris-Sorbonne, 2009), 63–81.

——, 'Portraits and afterlives: Diderot and Montaigne', in Holland, Anna and Scholar, Richard (eds), *Pre-Histories and Afterlives: Studies in Critical Method for Terence Cave* (London: Legenda, 2009), 95–105.

——, 'Pré-histoire d'un emblème des Lumières: l'aveugle-né de Montaigne à Diderot', in Moreau, Isabelle (ed), *Les Lumières en mouvement: la circulation des idées au XVIIIe siècle* (Lyon: ENS, 2009), 173–97.

——, 'Eyes Wide Shut: *Le Rêve de d'Alembert*', in Fowler, James (ed.), *New Essays on Diderot* (Cambridge: Cambridge University Press, 2011), 141–57.

——, 'Philosophy, Ethics and the Work of Fiction', in Tadié, Alexis and Scholar, Richard (eds), *Fiction and the Frontiers of Knowledge in Europe, 1500–1800* (Aldershot: Ashgate, 2011), 107–21.

Undank, Jack, *Diderot: Inside, Outside, and In-Between* (Madison, WI: Coda Press, 1979).

Undank, Jack, and Josephs, Herbert, *Diderot: Digression and Dispersion: A Bicentennial Tribute* (Lexington, KY: French Forum, 1984).

Vartanian, Aram, *Diderot and Descartes: A Study of Scientific Naturalism in the Enlightenment* (Princeton: Princeton University Press, 1953).

——, 'La Mettrie and Diderot Revisited: An Intertextual Encounter'. *Diderot Studies*, 21 (1983), 155–97.

Venturi, Franco, *Jeunesse de Diderot, 1713–1753* (Paris: Albert Skira, 1939).

Vernière, Paul, *Spinoza et la pensée française avant la révolution*, 2 volumes (Paris: Presses Universitaires de France, 1954).

Versini, Laurent, 'Diderot, piéton à Paris'. *Travaux de Littérature*, 13 (2000), 117–94.

Viala, Alain, *Lettre à Rousseau sur l'intérêt littéraire* (Paris: Presses Universitaires de France, 2005).

Volpilhac-Auger, Catherine, *Tacite en France de Montesquieu à Chateaubriand*. *SVEC*, 1993: 313.

Warman, Caroline, 'Intimate, Deprived, Uncivilised: Diderot and the Publication of the Private Moment', in Kahn, Andrew (ed.), *Representing Privates Lives of the Enlightenment*. *SVEC*, 2010: 11, 35–51.

Weygand, Zina, *The Blind in French Society from the Middle Ages to the Century of Louis Braille* (Stanford: Stanford University Press, 2009).

Williams, Wes, *Monsters and their Meanings in Early Modern Culture. Mighty Magic* (Oxford: Oxford University Press, 2011).

Yolton, John W., *Thinking Matter: Materialism in Eighteenth-Century Britain* (Oxford: Basil Blackwell, 1984).

Index

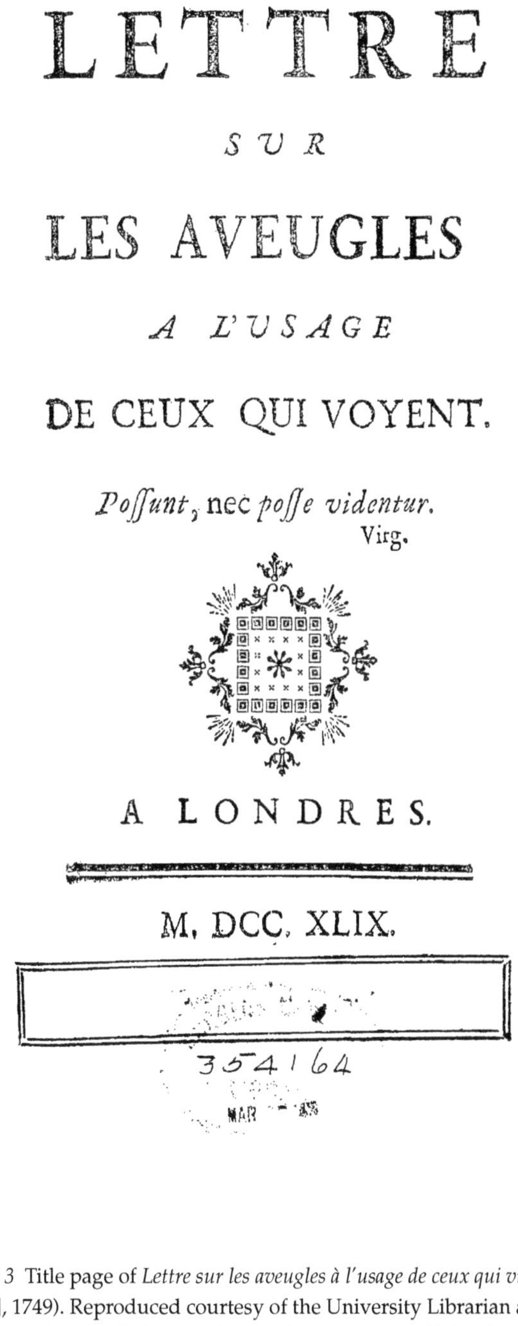

LETTRE

SUR

LES AVEUGLES

A L'USAGE

DE CEUX QUI VOYENT.

Possunt, nec *posse videntur.*
Virg.

A LONDRES.

M. DCC. XLIX.

Figure 3 Title page of *Lettre sur les aveugles à l'usage de ceux qui vient* (London [Paris], 1749). Reproduced courtesy of the University Librarian and Director, The John Rylands Library, The University of Manchester.

A

LETTER

ON

BLINDNESS

FOR THE

Use of those who have their SIGHT.

LONDON:
Printed for WILLIAM BINGLEY, at the Britannia,
No. 31, in Newgate-Street.
MDCCLXX.
[Price ONE SHILLING and SIX-PENCE.]

Figure 4 Title page of *A Letter on Blindness for the Use of those who have their Sight* (London, 1770). Reproduced courtesy of the University Librarian and Director, The John Rylands Library, The University of Manchester.

Appendix One

Denis Diderot, *Letter on the Blind for the Use of Those Who Can See* (1749)

Note on the Translation

This is the first English translation and edition of the *Lettre sur les aveugles* since the eighteenth century when it first appeared in 1770 as *A Letter on Blindness. For the Use of those who have their Sight* (see Figure 4).[1] That work was reprinted with some modifications and various appendices in 1780 and again in 1783 with the title, *An Essay on Blindness, in a Letter to a Person of Distinction.*[2] It also served as the basis for Margaret Jourdain's translation (1916),[3] which has recently been reproduced by David Adams in Denis Diderot, *Thoughts on the Interpretation of Nature and other Philosophical Works* (2000).[4]

Diderot was himself a translator of English into French and so is ***, who claims to have translated part of a fictitious work from English, the

1 *A Letter on Blindness. For the Use of those who have their Sight* (London: printed for William Bingley, at the Britannia, No. 31, in Newgate Street, 1770). Yvon Belaval and Robert Niklaus claim that there were three translations, dating from 1754, 1762 and 1780 (DPV, 4, p. 10). I can find no evidence of the first two of these. For that of 1780, see note 2.

2 *An Essay on Blindness, in a Letter to a Person of Distinction; Reciting the most interesting Particulars relative to Persons born Blind and those who have lost their Sight. Being an Enquiry into the Nature of their Ideas, Knowledge of Sounds, Opinions concerning Morality and Religion, &c. Interspersed with several anecdotes of Sanderson, Milton, and others. With copper-plates elucidating Dr. Sanderson's method of working geometrical problems. Translated from the French of M. Diderot, Physician to His most Christian Majesty* (London: printed for Richard Dymott opposite Somerset-House, in the Strand, 1773). A second edition of this work appeared in London, probably in 1780, printed for J. Barker, No. 7, Little Russell-Court, Drury-Lane.

3 *The Letter on the* Blind, in *Diderot's Early Philosophical Works*, Margaret Jourdain (trans. and ed.) (Chicago and London: The Open Court, 1916), pp. 68–141. Jourdain states: 'This translation has been collated with an eighteenth-century translation, undated and anonymous, entitled *A Letter on Blindness*', p. 141.

4 See Denis Diderot, *Thoughts on the Interpretation of Nature and other Philosophical Works*, David Adams (intro. and ann.) (Manchester: Clinamen, 2000), pp. 149–90.

Life and Character of Dr Nicholas Saunderson, supposedly written by one William Inchlif Esq. *** observes that readers who are able to read the work in the original, 'y remarqueront un agrément, une force, une vérité, une douceur qu'on ne rencontre dans aucun autre récit, et que je ne me flatte pas de vous avoir rendus, malgré tous les efforts que j'ai faits pour les conserver dans ma traduction' [will remark in it a certain something that is charming, powerful, true and gentle, which is to be found in no other tale and which I do not flatter myself to have rendered for you, in spite of all the efforts I have made to preserve it in my translation]. ***'s claim is ironic, not least because it would seem that there is no real original to which the reader could compare his translation.[5] That is not the case for the readers of my translation and so the sentiments that *** expresses ironically are ones that I wish to express here for real.

The two footnotes are Diderot's, as is the Index. The endnotes are mine and have been kept to a minimum. Where the *Letter* makes reference to other works of the period, the endnotes refer, where available, to the standard English translation. Names are given in their modern spelling (e.g. 'Puiseaux' for 'Puisaux', 'Molyneux' for 'Molineux') or have been corrected (e.g. 'Raphson' for 'Rapson', 'Saunderson' for 'Saounderson'). The six plates are reproduced by courtesy of the University Librarian and Director, The John Rylands University Library, The University of Manchester.

5 See above, p. 45.

Letter on the Blind for the Use of Those Who Can See

Possunt, nec *posse videntur*[1]

(London, 1749)[2]

I had my doubts, Madame, about whether the blind girl whose cataracts Monsieur de Réaumur[3] has just had removed, would reveal to you what you wanted to know, but it had not occurred to me that it would be neither her fault nor yours. I have appealed to her benefactor in person and through his best friends, as well as by means of flattery, but to no avail, and the first dressing will be removed without you. Some highly distinguished people have shared with the philosophers the honour of being snubbed by him. In a word, he only wanted to perform the unveiling in front of eyes of no consequence.[4] Should you be curious to know why that talented Academician makes such a secret of his experiments, which cannot, in your view, have too many enlightened witnesses, I should reply that the observations of such a famous man do not so much need spectators while they are being performed as an audience once the performance is over. So, Madame, I have returned to my initial plan, and having no choice but to miss out on an experiment which I could not see would be instructive for either you or me, but which will doubtless serve Monsieur de Réaumur rather better, I began philosophizing with my friends on the important matter that it concerns. How delighted I should be were you to accept the account of one of our conversations as a substitute for the spectacle that I so rashly promised you!

The very day that the Prussian[5] was performing the cataract operation on Simoneau's daughter,[6] we went to question the man-born-blind of Puiseaux.[*] He is a man not lacking in good sense and with whom many people are acquainted. He knows a bit of chemistry and followed the botany lessons in the King's Garden quite successfully.[7] His father taught philosophy to much acclaim in the University of Paris and left him an honest fortune, which would easily have been enough to satisfy his remaining senses had his love of pleasure not led him astray in his youth. People took advantage of his inclinations, and he retired to a little town in the provinces whence he comes to Paris once a year, bringing with him liqueurs of his own distillation, which are much appreciated. There you have, Madame, some details which, though not very philosophical, are for that very reason all the more suitable for persuading you

---

* Small town in the Gâtinais.

that the character of whom I am speaking is not imaginary.[8]

We arrived at our blind man's house around five o'clock in the evening to find him using raised characters to teach his son to read. He had only been up for an hour, since, as you know, the day begins for him as it ends for us. His custom is to work and see to his domestic affairs while everyone else is asleep. At midnight, there is nothing to disturb him and he disturbs no one. The first task he undertakes is to put back in its place everything that has been moved during the day, and his wife usually wakes up to a tidy house. The difficulty the blind have in finding things that have been mislaid makes them fond of order, and I have noticed that people who are well acquainted with them share this quality, either owing to their good example or out of a feeling of empathy that we have for them. How unhappy the blind would be without the small acts of kindness of those around them! And how unhappy we would be too! Grand gestures are like large gold and silver coins that we rarely have any occasion to spend, but small gestures are the ready currency we always have to hand.

Our blind man is a very good judge of symmetry. Between us, symmetry is perhaps a pure convention, but between a blind man and the sighted, it is certainly so. By using his hands to study how the parts of a whole must be arranged such that we call it beautiful, a blind man can manage to apply this term correctly, but when he says *that's beautiful*, he is not judging it to be so; he is simply repeating the judgement of the sighted. And is that any different to what three quarters of people do when they judge a play they have listened to or a book they have read? To a blind man, beauty is nothing more than a word when it is separated from utility, and with one less sense organ, how many things are there, the utility of which escapes him? Are the blind not to be pitied for deeming beautiful only what is good? So many wonderful things are lost on them! The only compensation for their loss is the fact that their ideas of beauty, though much less broad in scope than ours, it is true, are much more precise than those of the clear-sighted philosophers who have written long treatises on the subject.

Our blind man constantly talks about mirrors. You are right in thinking he does not know what the word 'mirror' means, and yet he will never place a mirror face down. He expresses himself with as much sense as we do about the qualities and defects of the organ he lacks, and though he does not attach any ideas to the terms he uses, he nonetheless has an advantage over most other men in that he never uses them incorrectly. He speaks so well and so accurately on so many things that are absolutely unknown to him, that conversing with him would undermine the inductive reasoning we all perform, though we have no idea why, which assumes that what goes on inside us is the same as what goes on inside others.

I asked him what he understood by a mirror: 'A machine,' he replied, 'that projects things in three dimensions at a distance from themselves if they are correctly placed in front of it. It is like my hand inasmuch as I mustn't place it to one side of an object if I want to feel it.' Had Descartes been born blind, he would, it seems to me, have congratulated himself on such a definition. Indeed consider, if you will, the subtlety with which he had to combine certain ideas in order to arrive at it. Our blind man knows objects only through touch. He knows on the basis of what other men have told him that it is by means of sight that we know objects just as they are known to him through touch. At least, that is the only notion he can have of sight. He also knows that we cannot see our own faces, though we can touch them. Sight, so he is bound to conclude, is a kind of touch that only applies to objects other than our faces and which are located at a distance from us. Moreover, touch only gives him the idea of three dimensions and so he will further believe that a mirror is a machine that projects us in three dimensions at a distance from ourselves. How many famous philosophers have employed less subtlety to arrive at notions that are equally false? How surprising must a mirror be for a blind man though? And he must have been even more astonished when we told him that there are other machines that enlarge objects and others still that, without duplicating the objects, make them change place, bring them closer, move them further away, make them visible and reveal their tiniest parts to naturalists' eyes, and that there are some that multiply objects by the thousand and others that seem to alter what they look like completely. He asked us hundreds of bizarre questions about these phenomena. For example, he asked if it was only people called naturalists who could see with a microscope, and whether astronomers were the only people who could see with a telescope, whether the machine that enlarges objects was larger than the object that makes them smaller, whether the one that brings them closer was shorter than the one that moves them further away, and he was completely unable to understand how that other one of us who is, as he put it, repeated in three dimensions by the mirror, could elude the sense of touch. 'Here you have two senses', he said, 'that are made to contradict each other by means of a little machine. A better machine might perhaps make them agree with each other without the objects being any more real as a result; and perhaps a third, even better and less perfidious machine would make them disappear altogether and notify us of the error.'

'In your opinion, what are eyes?' Monsieur de . . . asked him. 'They are organs', replied the blind man, 'that are affected by the air in the same way as my hands are affected by my stick.' His reply took us aback, and as we stared at each other in wonder, he continued, 'That must be right because when I place my hand between an object and your eyes, you can see my hand but not the object. The same thing happens to me when I am looking for one thing with my stick and I come across something else instead.'

Madame, open Descartes' *Dioptrics* and there you will find the phenomena of vision related to those of touch, and optical plates full of men seeing with sticks.[9] Descartes and all those who have come after him have been unable to provide any clearer ideas of vision, and in this respect the great philosopher's superiority over our blind man was no greater than that of the common man who can see.

None of us thought to ask him about painting and writing, but it is clear that there is no question to which his comparison could not give a satisfactory answer, and I am in no doubt that he would have said that trying to read or see without eyes was like looking for a pin with a great big stick. We spoke to him only of those kinds of pictures that use perspective to give objects three dimensions and which are both so similar and so different to our mirrors, and we realized they confused as much as they confirmed his understanding of a mirror and that he was tempted to believe that since a mirror paints objects, a painter representing them would perhaps paint a mirror.

We saw him thread very small needles. Might I ask you, Madame, to look up from your reading here and imagine how you would proceed if you were he? In case you can't think how, I shall tell you what our blind man does. He places the needle long-ways between his lips with the eye of the needle facing outwards and then, sucking in with his

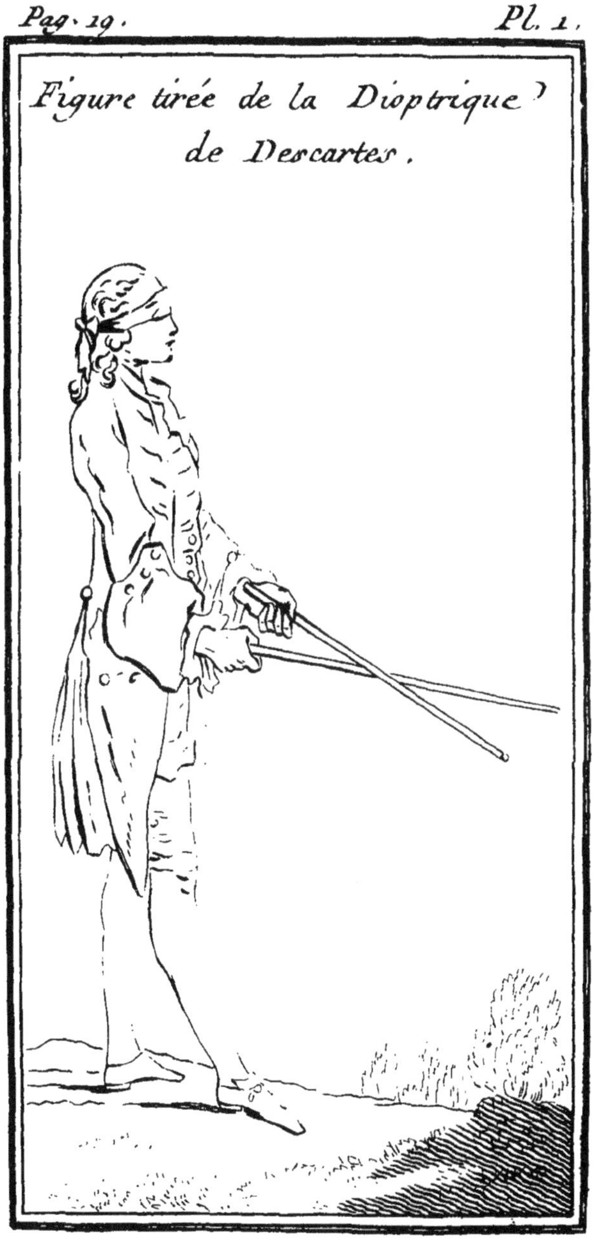
Pag. 19.
Pl. 1.
Figure tirée de la Dioptrique de Descartes.

tongue, he pulls the thread through the eye, except when it is too thick, but in that case someone who can see is in no less difficulty than someone who can't.

He has an amazing memory for sounds, and faces afford us no greater diversity than voices do him. They present him with an infinite scale of delicate nuances, which elude us because we do not have as much interest in observing them as the blind man does. Such nuances are like our own faces inasmuch as, of all the faces we have ever seen, the one we recall the least well is our own. We only study faces to recognize people, and if we cannot remember our own, it is because we will never be in the position of mistaking ourselves for someone else nor someone else for ourselves. Moreover, the way the senses work together prevents each one from developing on its own. This will not be the only time I shall make this observation.

On this matter, our blind man told us that he might have thought himself to be pitied for lacking our advantages and have been tempted to see us as superior beings, had he not on hundreds of occasions felt how much we deferred to him in other ways. This remark prompted us to make another. This blind man, we said to ourselves, has as high a regard for himself as he does for those of us who can see, perhaps even higher. Why then if an animal has reason, which we can hardly doubt, and if it weighed up its advantages over those of man, which it knows better than man's over it, would it not pass a similar judgement? He has arms, the fly might say, but I have wings. Though he has weapons, says the lion, do we not have claws? The elephant will see us as insects; and while all animals are happy to grant us our reason, which leaves us in great need of their instinct, they claim to be possessed of an instinct, which gives them no need for our reason. We have such a strong tendency to overstate our qualities and underplay our faults that it would almost seem as though man should be the one to do the treatise on strength, and animals the one on reason.

One of us decided to ask our blind man whether he would like to have eyes. He replied, 'If I wasn't so curious, I'd just as well have long arms, as it seems to me that my hands could teach me more about what's happening on the moon than your eyes or telescopes can, and besides, eyes stop seeing well before hands stop touching. It would be just as good to improve the organ I already have, as to grant me the one I lack.'

Our blind man locates noises or voices so accurately that I have no doubt that, with practice, blind people could become highly skilled and highly dangerous. I shall tell you a story that will convince you how wrong we would be to stay still were he to throw a stone at us or fire a pistol, regardless of how little practice he might have had with a firearm. In his youth, he had a fight with one of his brothers who came out of it very badly. Angered by some unpleasant remarks that his brother directed at him, he seized the first object that came to hand, threw it at him, hit him right in the middle of his forehead and laid him out on the ground.

This affair and some others made him known to the police. The visible signs of authority that affect us so powerfully do not impress the blind. Our blind man appeared before the magistrate as if before his equal. Threats did not intimidate him. 'What will you do to me?' he asked Monsieur Hérault.[10] 'I shall throw you in the dungeon', replied the magistrate. 'Oh, Sir,' replied the blind man, 'that's where I've been for twenty-five years.' What a reply, Madame! And what a line for a man who likes moralising as much as I do! We depart this life as though it were an enchanting spectacle, whereas the blind man departs it as though it were a prison, and although we enjoy living more than he does, you must agree he has many fewer regrets in dying.

The man-born-blind of Puiseaux works out how close he is to the fire by how hot it is, how full a receptacle is by the sound liquid makes as he decants it, and how near he is to other bodies by the way the air feels on his face. He is so sensitive to the most minor changes in the atmosphere that he can tell a street from a cul-de-sac. He can guess with astonishing accuracy how much something weighs and how much a bottle can hold, and his arms make such precise scales and his fingers such experienced compasses that, in matters of statics, I would always back our blind man against twenty sighted people. The surface of the skin is no less subtly differentiated to him than the sound of the voice, and there is no reason to fear that he might mistake his wife for another woman, unless he stood to gain by it. It would very much appear, however, that in a land of the blind, either wives would be communal or its adultery laws would be very strict. It would be very easy for wives to deceive their husbands by using a sign they had agreed with their lovers.

He judges beauty by touch. That is understandable, but what is not so easy to grasp is that he also bases his judgement on the sound of a person's voice and the way they pronounce words. We would need an anatomist to explain whether there is some relationship between the parts of the mouth and palate and the external shape of the face. He can make little things by turning them on a lathe and do small pieces of needlework; he can level using a set square; he can take ordinary machines apart and put them back together; and he knows enough music to be able to play a piece if he is told the notes and their relative values. He is able to judge the duration of time much more precisely than we can by the sequence of actions and thoughts. The beauty of someone's skin, their firm, plump curves, the sweet smell of their breath and the charming sound of their voice and diction are qualities by which he sets great store.

He married so as to have eyes of his own. He had previously intended to marry a deaf woman who would have lent him her sight and to whom he would have lent his hearing.[11] Nothing surprised me so much as his singular ability to do a great number of things, but when we revealed our surprise, he said: 'It is clear to me, Gentlemen, that you are not blind, since you are surprised at what I can do. So why aren't you also amazed that I can speak?' There is, I believe, more philosophy in that reply than he intended. It is surprising how easily we learn to speak. We only succeed in attaching an idea to a large number of terms that cannot be represented by sensible objects and which have, as it were, no body, by means of a series of subtle and profound analogies which we perceive between these non-sensible objects and the ideas they excite in us. As a result, we must admit that a blind man is bound to find it more difficult to learn to speak, since the number of non-sensible objects is much greater for him than it is for other people, and so he has much less scope for comparing and combining. How can we expect the word 'physiognomy', for example, to become fixed in his memory? It is a charming kind of quality consisting of things that are so barely perceptible to a blind man and hardly more so to those of us who can see, that we would have great trouble saying exactly what it is to be possessed of a physiognomy. If it is in the eyes, touch is unable to grasp it; and in any case, what are blank eyes, lively eyes, intelligent eyes, etc. to a blind man?

From this, I conclude that we are well served by the ways in which our different senses and sense organs cooperate. But it would be a very different thing if we exercised each one separately and never used two together when one on its own would suffice. To add touch to sight when the eyes are sufficient on their own is like taking two already very lively horses and harnessing a third to them at ninety degrees so that one pulls in one direction while the other two pull in the other.

Since I have never doubted the great influence of our senses and organs on our metaphysics and morals, nor that our most purely intellectual ideas, if I may call them that, are closely related to the organisation of our bodies, I began to ask our blind man about vice and virtue. First I learnt that he had an extraordinary aversion to theft, which was caused in him by two things: the ease with which other people could steal from him without him noticing and, perhaps even more importantly, the ease with which they could see him stealing from them. It's not that he doesn't know perfectly well how to guard himself against the additional sense he knows us to have nor that he is unaware of how best to cover up a theft. He sets little store by modesty. If it weren't for the protection they afforded from draughts, he could hardly comprehend why we wear clothes, and he openly admits to being unable to work out why we cover one part of our bodies rather than others, and is even less able to grasp our bizarre practice of covering particular parts of the body, whose functions, combined with the disorders to which they are prone, ought to require them to be kept free. Although we live in a century in which the philosophical spirit has rid us of a great number of prejudices, I don't think we will ever go so far as to misunderstand the prerogatives of modesty quite as completely as my blind man. To him, Diogenes would not have been a philosopher.[12]

Since of all the external signs that evoke ideas of sympathy and pain in us, the blind are only affected by the sound of suffering, I suspect them, in general, of being inhumane. What difference can there be for a blind man between a man urinating and a man shedding blood without a whimper? Don't we too stop sympathising when something is so far away or so small that we can't see it any more clearly than a blind man can? How dependent virtue is on our way of feeling and on the degree to which we are affected by external things! Consequently I don't doubt that, were it not for the fear of punishment, many people would find it less difficult to kill a man, were he far enough away that he looked as small as a swallow, than to kill a bull with their bare hands. If we feel compassion for a horse in pain and squash an ant without giving it a moment's thought, are we not following the same principle? Madame, how different blind morality is to ours! And how different again a deaf man's is to a blind man's, and how imperfect, to say the least, would our morality seem to a being who had one more sense than we do!

Our metaphysics are no more in line with theirs. How many of our principles are absurd to the blind, and vice versa! I could go into detail about that here, which would no doubt be to your amusement, but some people who see crime everywhere would have no hesitation in accusing me of irreligion, as though it were down to me to make the blind perceive things in a manner other than that in which they perceive them. I shall be content to make one observation with which I believe everyone must agree, namely that the grand argument that is derived from nature's marvels is very weak for the blind. The ease with which we create, as it were, new objects by means of a little mirror is something more incomprehensible to them than the stars, which they have been condemned never to see. That luminous globe that moves from east to west is less astonishing to them than a little fire which they can increase or decrease at their own convenience, for since they see matter in a much more abstract way than we do, they are less unlikely to believe it can think.

If a man who had only been able to see for a day or two were to find himself lost in a land of the blind, he would have to decide between keeping quiet and being taken for a madman. Every day he would proclaim some new mystery, which would only be a mystery to the blind and which the freethinkers would pride themselves on not believing. Could the defenders of religion not make good use of such stubborn and, to some extent, such fair and yet such ill-founded unbelief? If you entertain that supposition for a moment, it will bring to mind in another guise the history and persecutions of those who were unlucky enough to discover the truth in the dark ages and unwise enough to reveal it to their blind contemporaries, among whom they had no crueller enemies than those whose order and education ought, it seemed, to have made them hold the least dissimilar views.

So I leave behind the morality and metaphysics of the blind and move on to less important things, though they are more closely related to the point of all the observations people are constantly making ever since the Prussian arrived. Question one: how does a man-born-blind form ideas of shapes? I think he gains the idea of a line by moving his hands from one place to the next and feeling a body pass continuously through his fingers. If he slides his fingers along a taught thread, he gains the idea of a straight line, and by following the curve of a slack thread, he gains the idea of a curved line. More generally, it is from repeated experiences of touch that he acquires the memory of the sensations he had at different points, and since he is able to combine these sensations or points, he can form shapes. A straight line for a blind man who is not a geometer is nothing other than the memory of a series of sensations of touch arranged in the same way as a taut piece of string, and a curved line the memory of a series of sensations of touch as they relate to the surface of some concave or convex body. With practice, a geometer is able to rectify these lines by working out their properties, but geometer or no, the man-born-blind relates everything to his fingertips. We combine coloured points, whereas he only combines palpable points or, to be more precise, the sensations of touch that he can remember. Nothing happens in his head the way it does in ours because he cannot imagine, since to imagine you must colour in a background and make some points stand out against it by supposing them to be of a different colour. If you make the points the same colour as the background, they immediately merge together and the shape disappears; at least, that's how things happen in my imagination and I presume other people don't imagine any differently. So when I decide to perceive a straight line in my head other than by means of its geometrical properties, I begin by stretching out a white canvas, on which I pick out a series of black points that are all arranged in a line. The stronger the colour of the backdrop and the colour of the points, the more clearly I perceive them, and a shape in a colour that is very similar to that of the background is no less tiring to contemplate in my imagination than outside my head and on a canvas.

So you see, Madame, it would be possible to come up with some simple rules for imagining several objects of several different colours at the same time, but such laws would be of no use whatsoever to a man-born-blind. Since he is unable to imagine colour and, as a result, unable to make shapes in the way we understand, he has no memory of anything other than the sensations gained through touch, which he relates to different points, places or distances, and out of which he makes shapes. It is so uniformly the case that we do not make shapes in our imagination other than by colouring them, that if we were asked to touch little spheres in the dark, we would immediately suppose them to be black or white or some other colour, and if we did not suppose them to be any colour, we would be like the man-born-blind and have nothing more than the memory of little sensations at our fingertips that would be consistent with those produced by small round bodies. If this memory is very fleeting in us and we barely have any idea how a blind man grasps, remembers and combines the sensations of touch, it is because our eyes have put us in the habit of doing everything with colours in our imaginations. I have myself, however, had the experience of being in the grip of a violent passion and felt my whole hand tremble as the impressions of bodies that I had touched a long time ago were reawakened in me as vividly as if they were still present to my touch, and I could very clearly perceive an exact correlation between the outlines of my sensation and those of these absent bodies. Although sensation is indivisible in itself, it occupies, if I may put it like this, an extended space, which the man-born-blind is able to enlarge or reduce by making the affected area larger or smaller. In so doing, he composes points, surfaces and bodies, and he could even make a body as large as the earth's sphere, were he to suppose his fingertip as large as the sphere and feel its full height, width and depth.

I don't know what could more clearly demonstrate the existence of the inner sense[13] than that faculty, which is weak in us but strong in men-born-blind, and which enables us to feel or recall the sensations of bodies even when they are absent and no longer perceptible. We are unable to make a man-born-blind understand how our imaginations paint absent objects to us as though they were present, but we can very easily recognize in ourselves the faculty that makes us able to feel an absent body at our fingertips, just as a man-born-blind can. To achieve this effect, press your index finger and thumb together and close your eyes; separate your fingers and immediately examine what happens inside you afterwards, and tell me if the sensation does not last for a long while after you have stopped pressing down, and whether while that pressure persists, you feel as though your soul is more in your head or in your fingertips, and whether the pressure does not give you the feeling of a surface equal to the space occupied by the sensation. It is only on the basis of the strength or weakness of the sensory impression that we can tell the difference between the sensation of beings that are present outside us and their representation in our imaginations. Similarly, the man-born-blind can only tell the difference between the real presence of an object at his fingertips and the sensation of it, on the basis of the strength or weakness of that same sensation.

If a philosopher who was born blind and deaf were ever to come up with a man on Descartes' model, I dare say, Madame, he would place the soul in the fingertips because they are the source of his principal sensations and all of his knowledge.[14] And who would tell him that his head is the main seat of his thoughts? If our heads find the labours of the imagination exhausting, it is because the effort of imagining is quite similar to that of perceiving objects that are very close to us or very small. But it is not like that for the man-born-blind-and-deaf, since the sensations he gains from his touch form, as it were, the cast of all his ideas, and so I would not be surprised if thinking deeply left his fingertips as tired as it does our heads. I would not be concerned by a philosopher objecting that the nerves are the cause of our sensations and that they all start at the brain, because even if he were to demonstrate those two propositions with a clarity to match their present lack of it, the blind man would need only to be told of all the things that doctors have dreamt up on the subject and he would hold onto his own opinion.[15]

Yet if a blind man's imagination is nothing other than the faculty of recalling and combining the sensations of palpable points, and that of a man who can see, the faculty of recalling and combining visible or coloured points, it follows that the man-born-blind perceives things in a much more abstract manner than we do, and that when it comes to questions of pure speculation, he is perhaps less prone to error than we are, since abstraction consists simply of mentally separating the sensible qualities of bodies either from each other or from the body that underlies them, and errors are made when that separation has either been performed in the wrong way or at the wrong stage; in the wrong way when it's a question of metaphysics, and at the wrong stage when it's a question of physico-mathematics.[16]

One way that is almost guaranteed to produce an error in metaphysics is not to make the objects in question as simple as possible, and the secret to obtaining a wrong answer in physico-mathematics is to suppose the objects to be less complex than they are.

There is one kind of abstraction of which so few men are capable that it seems to be reserved for pure intellects. It is one that reduces everything to numerical units. Everyone must agree that the results of this kind of geometry would be very accurate and that its formulas would be very general, since there are no objects, either real or possible, that such simple units cannot represent, be they points, lines, surfaces, solids, thoughts, ideas, sensations, and . . . if, by chance, this was the basis for Pythagoras's doctrine,[17] we could say of him that he failed in his project because that kind of philosophizing is too far beyond us and much closer to that of the Supreme Being who, according to the ingenious expression of an English geometer, is perpetually *geometrizing* in the universe.[18]

The pure and simple unit is too vague and too general a symbol for us. Our senses always bring us back to signs that are better suited to our mental capacity and physical organisation. We have even made these signs communal so that they can serve as a storehouse, so to speak, for the mutual commerce of our ideas. We have instituted some for the eyes, namely characters, and some for the ears, namely spoken sounds, but we have none for touch, even though there is a proper way of talking to this sense and of obtaining a reply. In the absence of this language, the channel of communication between men-born-deaf-dumb-and-blind and us is broken. They develop, but they remain feeble-minded. Perhaps they could acquire ideas if we could communicate with them as children and in a manner clearly defined and agreed, regularized and standardized; in short, if we were to draw the same characters on their hands as the ones we draw on paper, and if we were always to attach the same meaning to them.

Would this language not seem to you, Madame, to be as good as any other? In fact, does it not already exist? And could you swear that no one has ever used it to communicate anything to you? All we would need to do, if we found it too slow to use ordinary written characters to communicate through this sense, would be to formalize it and create a dictionary and grammar of it.

Knowledge has three points of entry into the soul, and we have blocked one of these up through lack of signs. Had we neglected the other two, we would have been reduced to the condition of animals. Just as squeezing tight is the only way we can communicate by touch, animal cries would have been our only means of aural communication. Madame, only someone who is deprived of a sense can understand the benefits of the symbols that are available to their remaining senses, and people who are unlucky enough to be deaf, dumb and blind or who come to lose these three senses in some accident would be delighted to have a clear and precise language for touch.

It is so much easier to use symbols that have already been invented than it is to be the inventor of them, as one has to be when they are lacking. How much better it would have been for Saunderson[19] if, at the age of five, palpable arithmetic had been waiting for him, instead of him having to invent it at the age of twenty-five! This Saunderson, Madame, is another blind man who is not irrelevant to our conversation. They say amazing things about him, and there is not a single one that is not to be believed on the basis of his achievements in literature and his talents in the mathematical sciences.[20]

He used the same machine for algebraic calculations as he did for the description of rectilinear shapes. You would not be displeased to have the machine explained to you, providing you could understand it, and you will see that it presupposes no knowledge you don't already have and you would find it very useful should you ever fancy feeling your way through some long calculations.[21]

Imagine a square, as shown in Plate II, divided into four equal parts by perpendicular lines going down the sides so as to give nine points, 1, 2, 3, 4, 5, 6, 7, 8, 9. Suppose this square had nine holes in it and you could put two kinds of pins in the holes, both of the same length and the same width, but one kind with a slightly larger head than the other.

The large-headed pins were only ever placed next to the centre of the square, while the small-headed ones were only ever placed on the sides, except in the case of the zero. The zero was marked by a large-headed pin placed in the centre of the little square with no other pin next to it. The number 1 was represented by a small-headed pin placed in the centre of the square with no other pin near it; the number 2 by a large-headed pin in the centre of

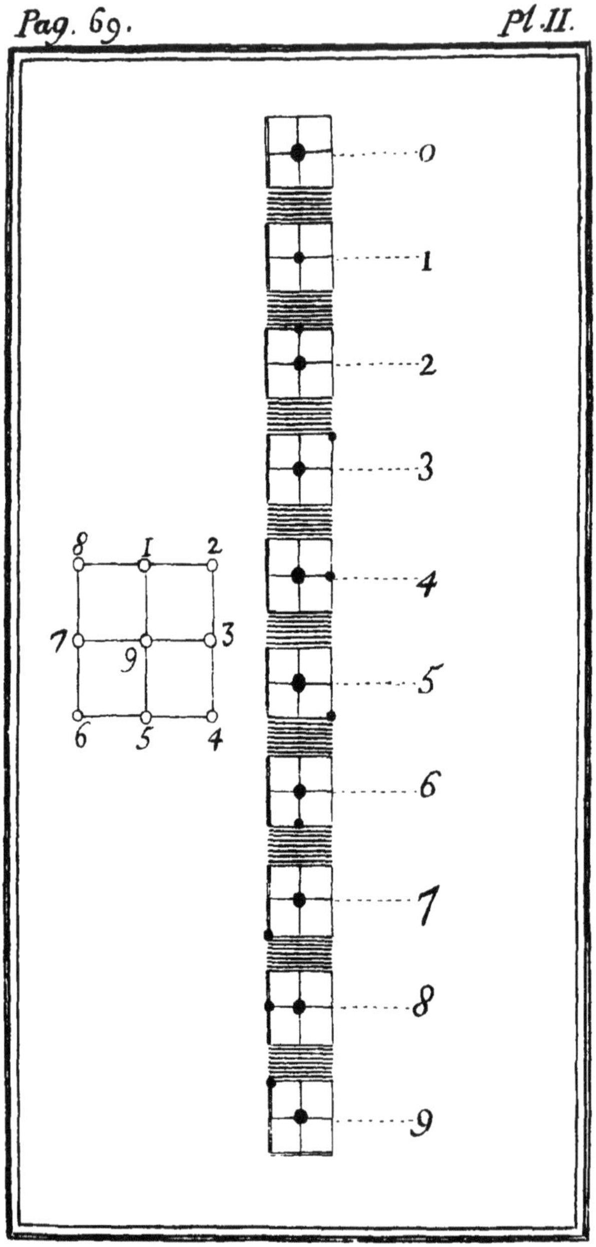
Pag. 69.
Pl. II.
8
1
2
7
9
3
6
5
4
0
1
2
3
4
5
6
7
8
9

the square with a small-headed pin to one side at point 1; the number 3 by a large-headed pin in the centre of the square with a small-headed pin to one side at point 2; the number 4 by a large-headed pin in the centre of the square with a small-headed pin to one side at point 3; the number 5 by a large-headed pin in the centre of the square with a small-headed pin to one side at point 4; the number 6 by a large-headed pin in the centre of the square with a small-headed pin to one side at point 5; the number 7 by a large-headed pin in the centre of the square with a small-headed pin to one side at point 6; the number 8 by a large-headed pin in the centre of the square with a small-headed pin to one side at point 7; the number 9 by a large-headed pin in the centre of the square with a small-headed pin to one side at point 8.

There you have ten different expressions accessible to touch, each corresponding to one of our arithmetical characters. Now imagine a table as large as you wish, divided into little squares arranged in a horizontal line and spaced at an equal distance apart, as shown in Plate III, and there you have Saunderson's machine.

You can easily understand that there is no number that cannot be written on that table, and that, as a result, no arithmetical operation that cannot be performed on it.

Suppose, for instance, that you wish to add up the following nine numbers and find out the total:

12345
23456
34567
45678
56789
67890
78901
89012
90123

I write them on the table as you say them to me, the first digit of the first number on the left and on the first square to the left of the first line; the second digit of the first number on the left and on the second square to the left of the same line and so on.

I put the second number on the second row of squares, units beneath units, tens beneath tens, etc.

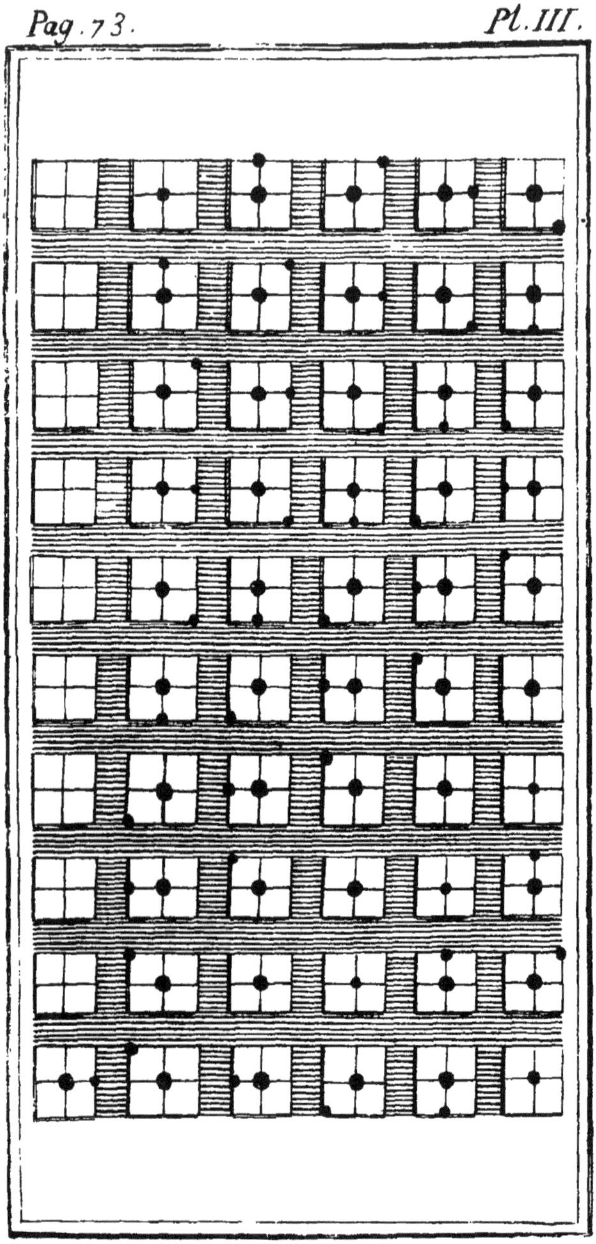
Pag. 73.
Pl. III.

I put the third number on the third row of squares and so on, as you see in Plate III. Then running my fingers down each row from top to bottom, starting with the one furthest to my left,[22] I add up the numbers expressed in that column, and write the remainder of the tens at the bottom. I move on to the second column to the left and work in the same way, and from that column to the next until I have completed the sum.

Here is how he used the same table to demonstrate the properties of rectilinear shapes. Supposing he was to demonstrate that parallelograms sharing a base and height also share a surface area, he would place his pins as shown in Plate IV. He would attach names to the corners and finish the demonstration with his fingers.[23]

Supposing Saunderson only used large-headed pins to mark the edges of his shapes, he could have arranged small-headed pins around them in nine different ways, all of which were familiar to him. Therefore he was only in difficulty in cases when the need to denominate a large number of corners in his demonstration forced him to have recourse to the letters of the alphabet.[24] We are not told how he used them.

We only know that he could run his fingers across his table with surprising agility, that he could successfully perform the longest of calculations, that he could stop and recognize when he had made a mistake, that he could check his work easily and that this task did not take him nearly as long as one might imagine, owing to the convenient way he prepared his table.

That preparation involved putting the large-headed pins in the centre of the square. Once he had done that, all he had left to do was decide on the value of the small-headed pins, except in those cases when he had to record a unit by putting a small-headed pin in the centre of the square in place of the large-headed one that was there before.

Sometimes, instead of marking a solid line with his pins, he would be content simply to put one pin at each corner or point of intersection, around which he would wind silk threads to create the edges of his shapes.[25] See Plate V.

He left behind some other machines that aided his study of geometry, but we don't know how exactly he used them, and it may require more wisdom to work it out than to solve any problem with integral calculus. Let some geometer try and explain to us what use he had for four pieces of solid

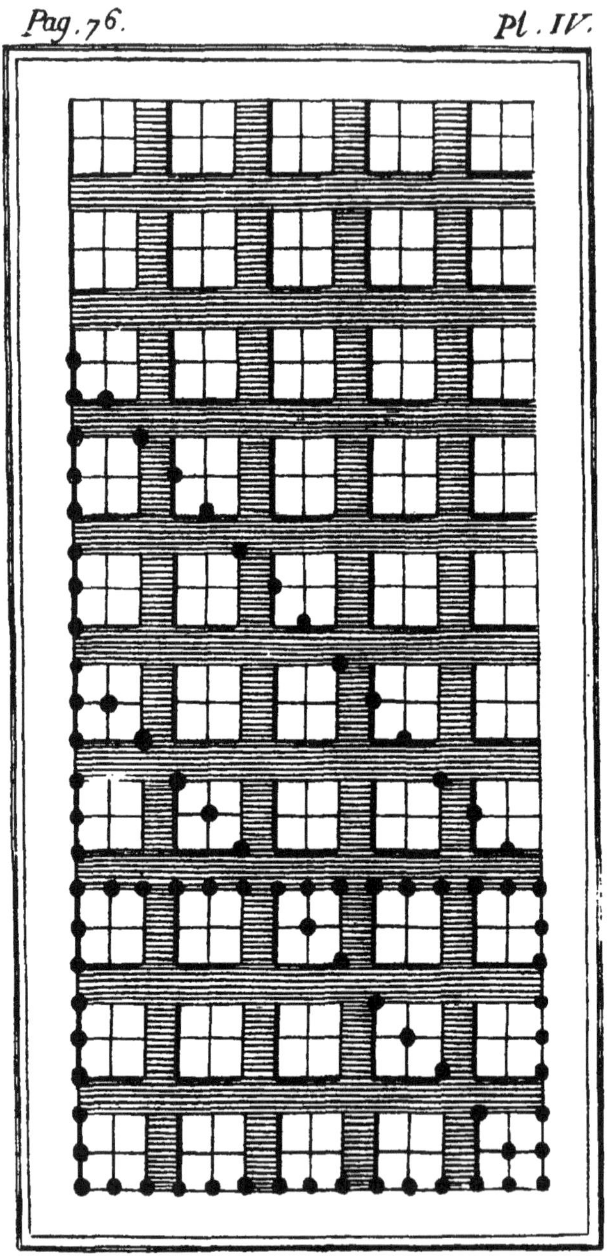

Pag. 79. Pl. V.

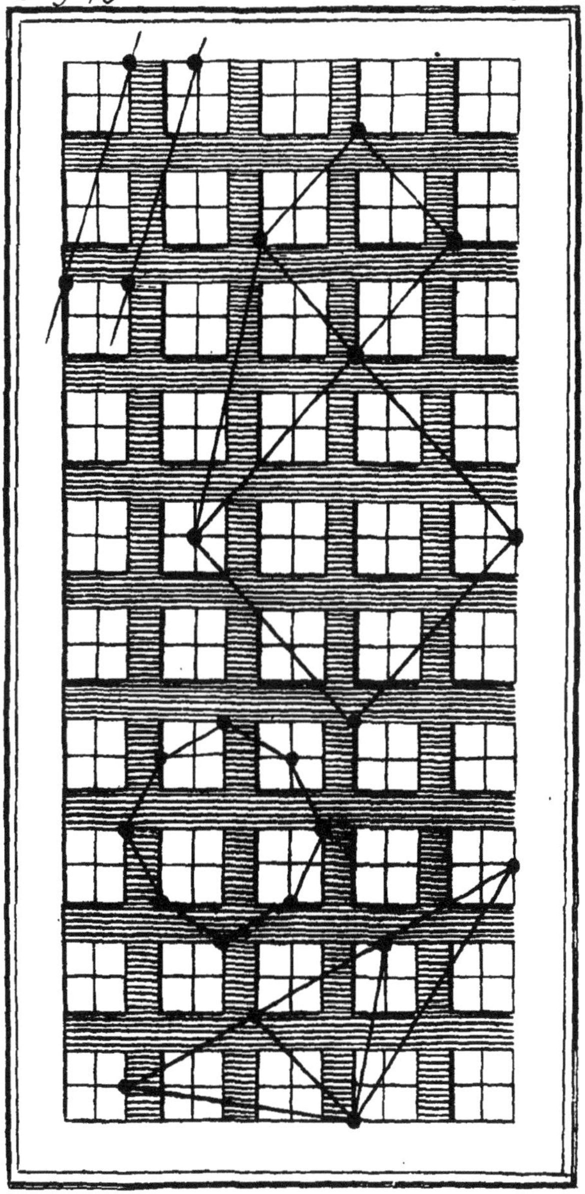

wood shaped like rectangular parallelepipeds, each one eleven inches long by five and a half wide and just over an inch thick, the opposite faces of which were divided into little squares similar to those of the abacus I have just described, except that they only had holes in places where the pins were pushed down as far as the head. Each surface showed nine arithmetical tables, each made up of ten numbers, and each of these ten numbers was made up of ten digits. Plate VI shows one of these little tables;[26] and here are the numbers it contained:

9 4 0 8 4
2 4 1 8 6
4 1 7 9 2
5 4 2 8 4
6 3 9 6 8
7 1 8 8 0
7 8 5 6 8
8 4 3 5 8
8 9 4 6 4
9 4 0 3 0

He is the author of an excellent work of its kind, the *Elements of Algebra*.[27] The only sign that he was blind is to be found in the singular nature of some of his demonstrations, which a man who can see might not have encountered before. It was he who first came up with the division of a cube into six equal pyramids, the points of which are at the centre of the cube with the bases forming each of its sides, and which is used in the simple mathematical proof that a pyramid is the third of a prism of the same base and height.

Saunderson's taste led him to study mathematics, and his poor fortune and his friends' advice obliged him to give public lessons. They were in no doubt that he would be better at it than he thought, owing to his prodigious talent for making himself understood. In fact, Saunderson spoke to his students as though it was they who were deprived of sight, but a blind man who expresses himself clearly to the blind must have much to gain from those who can see, since they have an extra telescope.

The people who wrote his biography say he was full of felicitous expressions and that seems very likely.[28] But what do you mean by felicitous expressions, you will perhaps ask? And I shall reply, Madame, that they are those that

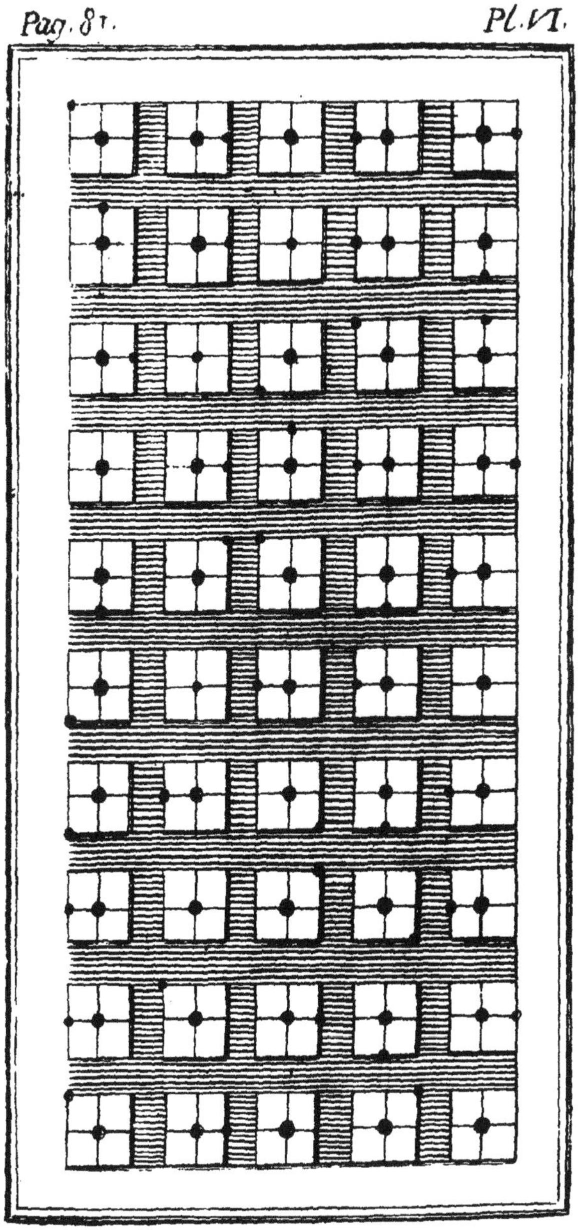

are appropriate to one sense, for instance, to touch, and at the same time metaphorical to another, such as sight, making them doubly enlightening for the listener, who can perceive both the true and direct light of the expression and the reflected light of the metaphor. Obviously on such occasions, Saunderson, extremely clever though he was, could only half understand himself because he could only perceive half the ideas that were attached to the terms he was using. Yet who doesn't find himself from time to time in the same situation? Such a mishap is common to idiots who occasionally crack excellent jokes, and to the cleverest of people who sometimes let slip a stupid remark, and neither realize what they have said.

I have noticed that a paucity of words also produces the same effect on foreigners who are not yet familiar with the language; they are obliged to say everything using a very small number of words, which obliges them to place some of them most felicitously. Yet languages in general lack suitable words for writers with lively imaginations, and so they find themselves in the same position as the foreigners with quick wits; the situations they invent, the subtle nuances they perceive in characters and the simplicity of the pictures they have to draw constantly lead them away from ordinary ways of speaking and make them adopt turns of phrase that are admirable as long as they are neither precious nor obscure, qualities we forgive more or less easily depending how much more wit and how much less knowledge of the language we have than they do. That is why, of all French writers, Monsieur de M . . .[29] is the one the English love most, and why Tacitus is the Latin writer whom *Thinkers* hold in the highest esteem.[30] The linguistic liberties they take pass us by, and we are struck only by the truth of the terms.

Saunderson was astonishingly successful at teaching mathematics at the University of Cambridge. He gave lectures on optics and the nature of light and colour; he explained the theory of vision; he wrote on the effects of lenses, the phenomena that produce rainbows, and many other subjects related to vision and the eye.

These facts will appear much less marvellous, Madame, once you realize there are three things that must be taken into consideration in any question that combines physics and geometry, namely the physical phenomenon that is to be explained, the suppositions that have been made by the geometer and the calculation that is done on the basis of those suppositions. It is obvious that however perspicacious the blind man may be, light and colour are unknown phenomena to him. He will be able to understand the suppositions because they relate to palpable causes, but he will be unable to grasp why the geometer supposed some things rather than others, for to do so, he would have to be able to compare the suppositions with the phenomena. The blind man thus accepts the suppositions as he finds them: a ray of light is a thin and elastic thread or a series of little bodies that strike our eyes at incredible speed, and he does his calculations on that basis. Physics turns into geometry, and the question becomes purely mathematical.

But what are we to make of the results of such calculations? 1. That they are sometimes extremely difficult to obtain, and that a physicist could happily come up with hypotheses that were as in keeping with nature as it was possible for them to be, but they would be worthless if he could not prove them geometrically, and that the greatest physicists, Galileo, Descartes, Newton, were therefore also great geometers; 2. That we derive more or less secure results from more or less complex initial hypotheses. When the calculation is founded on a simple hypothesis, the conclusions have the force of geometrical demonstrations; but when there are a large number of suppositions, the probability of each hypothesis being true diminishes, on the one hand, in proportion to the number of hypotheses, but increases, on the other, owing to the improbability of so many false hypotheses correcting each other accurately enough to obtain a result that is confirmed by the phenomena. Such a case would be the equivalent of a total sum being correct, though errors had been made in the partial sums of each of the numbers. It cannot be denied that such an outcome is possible, though you can see that it must be very unlikely all the same. The more numbers there are to be added together, the greater the likelihood that a mistake will have been made in each addition, but also the smaller the likelihood of a mistake if the result of the operation turns out to be correct. There is therefore one point at which the number of hypotheses is such that the calculation is as unlikely to be correct as it as possible to be. If A plus B plus C makes 50, shall I conclude from the fact that 50 is indeed the quantity of the phenomenon, that the suppositions represented by A, B and C were also correct? Not at all, for there are an infinite number of ways of reducing one of these letters and increasing the other two such that I still arrive at the answer 50, though the combination of three hypotheses is perhaps one of the most unfavourable.

One advantage of the calculus that I mustn't omit is that it excludes false hypotheses, because the result would contradict the phenomenon. If a physicist proposes to find the curve of a ray of light as it passes through the atmosphere, he is obliged make an assumption about the air density, the law of refraction, the nature and shape of light particles, and perhaps about some other essential elements too, which he does not include, however, either because he deliberately leaves them out or because they are unknown to him; he then works out the curve. If his calculation produces a result that contradicts nature, his suppositions were either incomplete or false. If the ray of light is described by the curve he produced, one of two things follows: either the suppositions have corrected themselves or they were correct. But which? He doesn't know, and yet that's the only thing he can be sure of.

I went through Saunderson's *Elements of Algebra* in the hope of finding out what I wanted to know from those who knew him well and had reported some details of his life, but my curiosity was not satisfied, and I imagined that an elements of geometry, after his fashion, would have been a more singular work on its own terms and much more useful for us. It would have given the definitions of point, line, surface, solid, angle, of intersections of lines and planes, using, I have no doubt, some highly abstract metaphysical principles close to those of the idealists. The name *Idealists* is given to those philosophers who are conscious only of their existence and of the sequence of sensations they experience inside themselves, and therefore admit nothing else. It is an extravagant system which could only, it seems to me, have been born of the blind and which, to the shame of the human mind and philosophy, is the most difficult to refute, though the most absurd of all. It is set out with as much sincerity as clarity in three *Dialogues* by Doctor Berkeley, Bishop of Cloyne.[31] The author of the *Essay on Human Knowledge*[32] should be invited to examine this work as it would give him the material for some useful, agreeable and subtle observations, in a word, for observations of the kind he does so well. It is well worth accusing him of idealism too, and this claim is liable to excite him owing less to its singularity than to the difficulty of refuting it according to his own principles, which are exactly the same as Berkeley's. According to them both and according to reason, the terms essence, matter, substance, substrate etc. offer the mind no insights. Furthermore, as the author of the *Essay* judiciously observes, whether we raise ourselves into the heavens or descend into the abyss, we never go beyond ourselves and it is only our own thought that we perceive.[33] Such is the conclusion of Berkeley's first dialogue and the very basis for his whole system. Would you not be curious to see these two enemies, whose weapons so closely resemble each other, take each other on? If one were to emerge victorious, it could only be the one who put them to the best use, but the author of the *Essay on Human Knowledge* has just written a *Treatise on Systems*,[34] in which he provides new evidence of the skill with which he wields his weapons and shows how formidable an adversary he is for systematic philosophers.

We're a long way from our blind men, I hear you say. But, Madame, you must be kind enough to allow me all these digressions, for I promised you a conversation, and I can't keep my promise unless you allow me this indulgence.

I read as attentively as I could what Saunderson had to say about infinity, and I can assure you that his ideas on that subject were very accurate and very clear, and that to him, most of our infinitesimalists would have been mere blind men. It will be up to you to judge for yourself, for although it is a difficult subject that takes you a little beyond your mathematical knowledge, with some preparation I should not despair of making it accessible to you and initiating you into that infinitesimal logic.

The example of this illustrious blind man proves that, with practice, touch can develop and become more sensitive than sight, since by running his hands over a series of medals, he could tell real from fake ones, despite the fact that the latter were forged convincingly enough to deceive a collector with a good eye.[35] He could also judge the precision of a mathematical instrument by feeling its markings with the very ends of his fingertips. Certainly those things are more difficult than judging how well a bust represents a person by touching it. All of this goes to show that a land of the blind could have its sculptors and could profit from statues in the same way we do, namely by preserving the memory of heroic actions and of people who were held dear. I have no doubt that the feelings they would have when they touched a statue would be even more powerful than the feelings we have when we look at one. How sweet it would be for a man who had been a very tender lover to run his hands over the charms he could recognize, and experience the illusion, which must work more powerfully on the blind than on the sighted, of them being brought back to life. Perhaps the greater the pleasure he would take in the memory though, the fewer regrets he would feel.

Saunderson shared with the blind man of Puiseaux the capacity to be affected by the most minor changes in the atmosphere and to perceive, particularly in calm weather, the presence of objects that were not more than a few paces away. It is said that one day he attended some astronomical observations that were being carried out in a garden, and the clouds, which from time to time hid the sun from view, caused a faintly perceptible change in the rays of light he could feel on his face, such that he could tell when the observations were possible and when they were not. You will perhaps be thinking that some disturbance occurred in his eyes to inform him whether it was light, but not whether objects were present or not, and I would have thought the same were it not for the certain fact that Saunderson was not only deprived of the sense of sight but also of its organ.

Saunderson's sight was in his skin. He had such an exquisitely sensitive epidermis that if a draughtsman were to sketch a friend's portrait on his hand, he would undoubtedly have been able, with a bit of practice, to recognize it and, feeling the sequence of sensations caused by the pencil, declare: 'It's Monsieur So and So'. There is therefore such a thing as painting for the blind: their own skin would be the canvas. These ideas are so far from being fanciful that I have no doubt that if someone drew Monsieur . . .'s little mouth on your hand, you would recognize it instantly. You must agree though that it would be even easier for a blind man to recognize it, despite the fact that you are used to seeing it and being charmed by it, because there are two or three things that enter into your judgement: the comparison between the painting done on your hand and the one deep inside your eye; the memory of the way you are affected by the things you feel and by the things you enjoyed seeing and admired; and finally, the application of this data to the question the draughtsman asks as he traces the outline of a mouth on your hand with the nib of his pencil, namely, 'Whose mouth am I drawing?' For a blind man, by contrast, the sum of the sensations produced by someone's mouth on his hand is identical to the sum of the sequence of sensations produced the draughtsman's pencil as he represents it.

I could add to the stories of the blind man of Puiseaux and Saunderson those of Didymus of Alexandria, Eusebius the Asiatic, Nicaise of Mechlin and some others who seemed to be so far above the rest of mankind despite having one fewer sense,[36] that poets might have said, without any exaggeration, that the gods were jealous and deprived them of a sense so as to have no equals among the mortals. For who was this Tiresias, who discovered the gods' secrets and had the power to see into the future, if he wasn't a blind philosopher, whose memory has come down to us through fable? But let's move no further away from Saunderson and follow this extraordinary man to the grave.

As he was nearing death, a very talented minister, Mr Gervaise Holmes,[37] was called to his bedside, and together they had a conversation about the existence of God, which has come down to us in fragments and which I will do my best to translate for you as they are well worth the trouble. The minister began by arguing in favour of nature's marvels; 'Ah Sir', replied the blind philosopher, 'forget that beautiful great spectacle that was never made for me! I have been condemned to live my life in darkness, and you cite wonders I can't understand and which are proof only for you and those who see as you do. If you want me to believe in God, you must make me touch him.'

'Sir,' the minister skilfully replied, 'run your hands over your own body and you will feel God in the admirable mechanism of your sense organs.'

'Mr Holmes,' Saunderson said, 'I repeat, all that is not as beautiful to me as it is to you. And even if the animal mechanism were as perfect as you claim, and I want to believe it is because you are an honest man and wholly incapable of deceiving me, what does it have in common with a supremely intelligent being? If you marvel at it, it might be because you tend to think anything that seems to be beyond your powers is a marvel. I have been the object of your wonder so often that I have a very low opinion of the things that amaze you. People have come to see me from all over England because they could not imagine how I was able to do geometry, which you must admit means that such people did not have a very clear notion of what is possible. If we think a phenomenon is beyond man, we immediately say it's God's work; our vanity will accept nothing less, but couldn't we be bit less vain and a bit more philosophical in what we say? If nature presents us with a problem that is difficult to unravel, let's leave it as it is and not try to undo it with the help of a being who then offers us a new problem, more insoluble than the first. Ask an Indian how the world stays up in the air, and he'll tell you that an elephant is carrying it on its back; and the elephant, what's he standing on? A tortoise. And that tortoise, what's keeping him up? . . . To you, that Indian is pitiful, yet one could say the same of you as you say of him. So, Mr Holmes, my friend, start by confessing your ignorance, and let's do without the elephant and the tortoise.'[38]

Saunderson paused for a moment; he seemed to be waiting for the minister to reply; but where can one attack a blind man? Mr Holmes took pride in the good opinion Saunderson had of his integrity and of the insights of Newton, Leibniz, Clarke and some other compatriots,[39] the world's foremost geniuses, all of whom had been struck by nature's marvels and recognized an intelligent being as its creator. There was no denying that this was his strongest argument against Saunderson. And the good blind man agreed that it would indeed be rash of him to deny what a man such as Newton had not found it beneath him to admit, but he explained nonetheless to the minister that Newton's testimony was not as powerful to him as that of the whole of nature had been to Newton, and that where Newton had taken God's word, he was reduced to taking Newton's.

'Consider, Mr Holmes', he added, 'how confident I have to be in what you and Newton say. I can't see anything and yet I will accept that everything is admirably ordered, but I am counting on you not demanding anything more of me. I defer to you as regards the current state of the universe in return for the freedom to think what I will about its ancient and primary state, to which you are no less blind than I am. You have no witnesses present that can testify against me, and in this respect your eyes are of no use to you. So you go on imagining, if you will, that the order that strikes you has always been in existence, but allow me to believe that nothing could be further from the truth, and that if we went back to the beginning of the universe and time,[40] and we felt matter start to move and chaos dissipate, for every couple of beings that were put together properly, we would encounter a multitude of shapeless ones. If I have no objection to your view of the present state of things, I can nonetheless question their former state. I can ask, for example, who told you all – you, Leibniz, Clarke and Newton – that when animals first came into being, there weren't some with no heads and others with no feet? I can claim that some had stomachs missing and others lacked intestines, that the ones with stomachs, teeth and palates, who looked as though they might survive, ceased to exist owing to some heart or lung defect, that monsters were wiped out one after another, that all defective combinations of matter disappeared and that the only ones to remain have mechanisms with no serious disorders, and can survive on their own and reproduce.

'On that basis, had the first man had a blocked larynx or not had suitable nourishment or had a problem with his reproductive organs, had he not met a mate or had he mated with another species, what would have happened to the human race then, Mr Holmes? It would have been swallowed up in the general purge of the universe, and that proud being called man would have been dissolved and scattered throughout the molecules of matter, and would have been and perhaps forever would have remained one of a number of possible outcomes.'

'Had there never been any shapeless beings, you would have no hesitation in saying that there never will be any and that I am indulging in fanciful hypotheses, but the order of the universe is not so perfect,' continued Saunderson, 'that monstrous outcomes are not produced from time to time.' And turning to the minister, he added, 'Look me in the face, Mr Holmes; I have no eyes. What have we done to God, you and I, such that one of us has that organ and the other is deprived of it?'[41]

Saunderson looked so deeply moved as he uttered these words that the minister and the rest of the gathering could not help feeling his pain and began to cry bitterly over him. The blind man noticed and said to the minister, 'Mr Holmes, I had heard about your goodness of heart and the evidence of it is very touching to me in my last moments, but if you hold me dear, do not deprive me in death of the consolation of knowing that I never caused anyone any pain.'

Then adopting a firmer voice once again, he added: 'It is therefore my conjecture that in the beginning when the universe was hatched from fermenting matter, my fellow men were very common. Yet couldn't my belief about animals also hold for worlds? How many lopsided, failed worlds are there that have been dissolved and are perhaps being remade and redissolved every minute in far away spaces, beyond the reach of my hands and your eyes, where movement is still going on and will keep going on until the bits of matter arrange themselves in a combination that is sustainable? Oh philosophers! Come with me to the edge of this universe, beyond the point where I can feel and you can see organised beings; wander across that new ocean with its irregular and turbulent movements and see if you can find in them any trace of that intelligent being whose wisdom you admire here.

'But why bother taking you out of your element? What is this world, Mr Holmes? It's a composite, subject to cycles of change, all of which exhibit a tendency towards destruction; a rapid series of beings that appear one after another, one replacing the next before vanishing; symmetry is fleeting, and order momentary. I criticized you a moment ago for judging the perfection of things by the standard of your own, and I could criticize you now for measuring how long things might last in relation to the length of your own life. You judge whether or not the world will continue to exist, in the same way the ephemeral fly judges whether or not you will. The world is eternal to you, just as you are eternal to the being that only lasts an instant. In fact, the insect is more reasonable than you are. What an amazing series of ephemeral lives it is, that stands as proof of your eternal life! How far that tradition stretches back! Yet we will all pass away without being able to determine either the actual area we occupied or the precise length of time we lasted. Time, matter and space may be only a single dot.'

Saunderson became more agitated in this conversation than his state of health would permit, and he went into a delirium lasting several hours,[42] from which he emerged only to exclaim, *'Oh God of Clarke and Newton, take pity on me!'* and die.

Thus Saunderson ended his days. You see, Madame, even all those arguments he had just put forward to the minister were not enough to reassure a blind man. It puts to shame those people whose arguments are no stronger than his but who are able to see and to whom the amazing spectacle of nature, from the rising of the sun to the setting of the tiniest stars, proclaims the existence and glory of its author! They have eyes, which Saunderson did not, and yet he had a purity of morals and an innocence of character that they lack. Thus they live their lives blind, and Saunderson dies as though he could see. The voice of nature can make itself heard clearly enough through his remaining organs, and his testimony will thereby be an even greater challenge to those who stubbornly shut their eyes and ears. I should willingly ask whether the true God was not more veiled to Socrates by the pagan darkness than he was to Saunderson, whose blindness deprived him of the spectacle of nature.

I am rather upset to discover, Madame, that other interesting details from the life of this illustrious blind man have not been passed down to us for your satisfaction as well as mine. There was perhaps more enlightenment to be had from his replies than from all the experiments that are currently being proposed. How very unphilosophical those who lived with him must have been! I make an exception for his disciple, Mr William Inchlif, who only saw Saunderson in his final moments and recorded his dying words, which I recommend anyone who can understand a little English to read in the original and which are contained in a work published in Dublin in 1747, entitled *The Life and Character of Dr Nicholas Saunderson, late Lucasian Professor of the Mathematics in the University of Cambridge. By his disciple and friend William Inchlif, Esq.*[43] They will remark in it a certain something that is charming, powerful, true and gentle, which is to be found in no other tale and which I do not flatter myself to have rendered for you, in spite of all the efforts I have made to preserve it in my translation.

Saunderson married the daughter of Mr Dickons, rector of Boxworth, in the county of Cambridge in 1713, and he had by her a son and a daughter who are still living.[44] His final farewell to his family is very touching: 'I am going,' he told them, 'where we all go. Spare me your distress, which I feel moved by. The signs of pain that escape your lips only make me more sensitive to the signs that elude my grasp. I feel no sorrow at leaving a life that has been nothing more to me than one long deprivation and endless yearning. Live as virtuously as I have and more happily, and learn to die as peacefully.' With that he took his wife's hand and held it tight in his for a while. Then he turned to face her as though trying to see her, blessed his children, embraced them all and begged them to withdraw as their presence was a crueller pain for his soul than the approach of death.

England is the country of philosophers, of the curious and the systematic, and yet without Mr Inchlif, all we would know of Saunderson is what the most ordinary of men would have told us, such as the fact that he could recognize places he had once visited by the sounds of the walls and the cobblestones, and a hundred other things of that sort, which he had in common with almost all other blind men. Is it common in England to meet blind men of Saunderson's merit, and is it an everyday occurrence to come across people who have never been able to see and who give lessons in optics?

People are trying to give sight to those born blind, but on closer examination, I think it would be found that philosophy has as much to gain by questioning a blind man of good sense. He would explain how things happen inside him, which could be compared to the way they happen inside us, and this comparison might solve all the problems that make the theory of vision and of the senses so complicated and so uncertain. However, I cannot, I confess, understand what it is hoped might be gained from a man who has just undergone a painful operation on a very sensitive organ that is disturbed by the slightest accident and often deceives those in whom it is healthy and who have enjoyed its benefits for some time. For my part, I would rather listen to a metaphysician familiar with the principles of physics, the elements of mathematics and the physical organisation of the body, lay out a theory of the senses, than to a man with no education and no knowledge and who had just acquired sight following a cataract operation. I should have less confidence in the responses of a man seeing for the first time than in the discoveries of a philosopher who had meditated long and hard on the matter in the dark or, to put it in poetic terms, had gouged out his eyes, the more comfortably to discover the workings of vision.[45]

If the experiments were to be at all reliable, the subject would need, at least, to have been be prepared for them a long time in advance, and have been brought up as and perhaps made into a philosopher, but making someone a philosopher cannot be done overnight, even when one is a philosopher oneself, and how long would it take if one were not? It takes even longer when one thinks one is. It would be most appropriate to wait a while after the operation before beginning the observations. To this end, the patient should be treated in darkness, his wounds must definitely have healed and his eyes must be healthy. I should not wish him to be exposed to daylight immediately; the glare of a bright light is blinding to us, so what must it be like to an extremely sensitive organ that has never received any sensory impressions to which it could have become accustomed?

But that's not all. It would still be very tricky to ensure that a subject who had been prepared in this way was put to good use and questioned subtly enough to make him explain precisely what was happening inside him. The questioning should be performed before a full Academy or rather, to ensure there were no superfluous spectators, only those people should be invited whose knowledge of philosophy, anatomy, etc. would make them deserving of an invitation. The most talented of men and the finest of minds would not be too good for it. Training and questioning a man-born-blind would have been a task not unfit for the combined talents of Newton, Descartes, Locke and Leibniz.

I shall finish this letter, which is already too long, with a question that was asked a long time ago. Thinking about Saunderson's singularity has made me see that it has never fully been answered. Suppose a man, born blind and now adult, who has been taught by his touch to distinguish between a cube and a sphere of the same metal and about the same size, so as when he felt one and the other, he could tell which was the cube, which the sphere.

It was Mr Molyneux who first asked this question and tried to answer it. He declared that the blind man would not be able to distinguish the sphere from the cube, 'for', he said, 'although he has learnt from experience in what manner the sphere and the cube affect his touch, he nonetheless does not yet know that what affects his touch in such or such a manner, must strike his eyes in such or such a fashion, nor that the protuberant angle of the cube that presses his hand in an uneven way must appear to his eyes as it does in the cube.'[46]

When Locke was consulted on this question, he said: 'I am entirely of Mr Molyneux's sentiment. I believe that the blind man would not be able, at first sight, to say with any confidence which is the cube and which the sphere if he only looked at them, although on touching them he could name them and distinguish them with certainty according to the difference in their shapes which he could recognize by his touch.'[47]

Monsieur l'abbé de Condillac, whose *Essay on Human Knowledge* was as pleasurable to read as it was useful, and whose excellent *Treatise on Systems* I am sending you along with this letter, has a particular sentiment in this matter.[48] There is no need to relate all the reasons he gives to support his argument, as that would be to deny you the pleasure of rereading a work in which his reasons are set out in such an agreeable and philosophical manner that it would be too risky for me to quote them out of context. I shall be content to observe that they all tend to demonstrate that the man-born-blind can either see nothing or see the cube and the sphere clearly, and that the condition, according to which the two bodies must be of the same metal and of about the same size, which it was judged necessary to include in the question, is incontestably superfluous for, so he might have said, if there is no essential relationship between the sensation of sight and that of touch, as Messrs Locke and Molyneux claim, they must agree that even a body that is two feet in diameter to the eye would disappear when it was touched. Monsieur de Condillac adds, however, that if the man-born-blind can see the bodies and distinguish the shapes, but nonetheless hesitates in his judgment of them, this can only be for some quite subtle metaphysical reasons that I shall explain to you in a moment.

So here we have two different sentiments on the same question, each belonging to a first-rate philosopher. It would seem that, having been discussed by men like Messrs Molyneux, Locke and the abbé de Condillac, there could be nothing left to say, but the same thing can be viewed from so many different angles that it wouldn't be surprising if they had not all been exhausted.

Those who have declared that the man-born-blind would be able to distinguish the cube from the sphere began by supposing a fact that is important to examine and which relates to whether or not a man-born-blind who had had his cataracts removed would be in a fit state to make use of his eyes in the moments immediately following the operation. They have simply said, 'As the man-born-blind compares the ideas of the sphere and the cube that he had gained by his touch with those he now gains by his sight, he will necessarily recognize that they are the same, and it would be bizarre to claim that it is the cube that gives him the idea of the sphere and that it is from the sphere that he gains the idea of the cube. He will therefore call cube and sphere what he called cube and sphere when he touched them.'

Yet what have their opponents argued in reply? They have also supposed that the man-born-blind would see as soon as his eyes were cured, and they have imagined that an eye that has had a cataract removed is like an arm that has recovered from paralysis. They claim that just as the latter does not need to exercise in order to have some feeling, so the eye does not either, and they add, 'Let us accord the man-born-blind a bit more philosophy than you did. Once he has reached the point in the argument where you left him, he will go a stage further and wonder who said that when I move towards the shapes and place my hands on them, they will not immediately undermine my expectations, the cube will not transmit the sensation of a sphere, and the sphere that of a cube? Only experience can teach me whether sight and touch relate to and agree with each other; these two senses could contradict each other without my knowing it; I might even believe that what I see is nothing but an appearance, had I not been told that these are the same bodies that I touched. It seems to me, in truth, that this one must be the one I was calling cube and that one, the one I was calling sphere. However, I am not being asked what seems to me to be the case, but rather what is the case, and I am simply not in a position to give a satisfactory answer to that last question.'

This line of thinking, so the author of the *Essay on the Origin of Human Knowledge* says, would be very confusing for the man-born-blind, and only experience can provide the answer. It would very much appear that Monsieur l'abbé de Condillac means to refer only to the experience that the man-born-blind would himself repeat by touching the bodies for a second time. You will sense in a moment why I am making this observation. That talented metaphysician could have added that a man-born-blind was obliged to think it all the less absurd that two senses might contradict each other, since that is what he thinks a mirror does, as I noted earlier.

Monsieur de Condillac goes on to observe that Mr Molyneux has confused the question by adding several conditions which can neither prevent nor remove the difficulties that metaphysics would present to the man-born-blind. This observation is all the more accurate since it is not out of place to assume the blind man to be acquainted with metaphysics, because in these philosophical questions, the experiment should always be done on a philosopher, that is, on a person who is able to grasp everything that his reason and the physical condition of his organs permit him to perceive in the questions being asked.

There, Madame, you have a summary of what has been said for and against this question; and in my examination of it, you will see how far those people who declared the blind man would see the shapes and distinguish the bodies were from realizing they were right, and how right those people who denied it were to think they were not wrong.

If we consider the question of the man-born-blind in more general terms than Mr Molyneux did, we can see that it involves two other questions, which we are going to consider in turn. It is possible to ask 1. whether the man-born-blind will see immediately after the cataract operation has been performed; 2. should he be able to see, whether he will be able to do so well enough to distinguish the shapes, whether he will be able, with any certainty, to give them the same names as he gave them when he touched them, and whether he will be able to prove that those are the right names.

Will the man-born-blind see immediately after his eyes have been treated? Those who claim that he won't be able to, say, 'As soon as the man-born-blind is possessed of the faculty of sight, the whole scene he has in front of him will enter and paint itself on the inside of his eyes. This image, which is made up of an infinite number of objects assembled in a very small space, is nothing but a confused mass of different shapes that he will be unable to tell apart. It is almost certainly the case that only experience can teach him how to judge the distance of objects and that he needs to move towards them, touch them, move back again, move towards them and touch them again in order to be sure that they are not part of him, that they are foreign to his being and that he is sometimes close to them and sometimes far away from them. Yet why should experience not also be necessary for him even to perceive them? Without experience, someone who perceives objects for the first time ought to think that when they move away from him or he so far away from them so that he can no longer see them, they stop existing, since it is only the experience of perceiving objects that do not move and of discovering that they remain where we left them that can tell us they continue to exist in our absence. It is perhaps for this reason that children are so readily consoled for toys that have been taken away. We cannot say they forget them readily since, if we consider that there are children aged two and half who know a considerable number of words and find it easier to remember a word than to say it, it is obvious that memory is strongest in childhood.

Wouldn't it be more natural to suppose that children think that things they can no longer see no longer exist, especially since their joy seems to be mixed with surprise when objects that were lost from view reappear. A nanny can help them acquire the idea of absent things by playing a little game with them in which she covers her face and suddenly uncovers it again. In this way, their experience teaches them a hundred times in a quarter of an hour that what ceases to be visible does not cease to exist. Whence it follows that it is experience that teaches us the notion of the continued existence of objects, that it is through touch that we acquire the idea of distance, that the eye may have to learn to see just as the tongue learns to talk, that it would not be surprising if one sense needed the help of another, and that touch, which guarantees the existence of objects outside ourselves when we see them, is perhaps the only sense able to tell us not, I think, what shape or other modifications objects may have, but simply that they are there.'

Added to these arguments are Cheselden's famous experiments.* The young man, whose cataracts this talented surgeon removed, could not for a long time see size, distance, location or even shape. An object the size of his thumb, placed in front of his eye to hide a house from view, seemed to him to be as large as the house. All objects felt as thought they were on his eyes, and they seemed to him to be touching the organ of sight in the same way that objects touched his skin. He could not tell the difference between something he judged to be round with his hands and something he judged to be angular by his sight, nor could he tell just by looking whether what he felt to be high or low was, in fact, high or low. He managed, though not without difficulty, to perceive that his house was larger than his room, but he was unable to conceive how it could be that his eye gave him that idea. He needed to repeat the same experience many times before he could be sure that paintings represented solid bodies, and having repeatedly looked at paintings and become convinced that he was not just seeing flat surfaces, he came to touch them with his hands and was most surprised to discover a single plane with no relief to it all, and he asked which was the lying sense, touch or sight? Paintings had the same effect on savages the first

* See *Elements of Newton's Philosophy* by Monsieur de Voltaire.[49]

time they saw them; they took painted figures to be living men, asked them questions and were astonished to receive no reply. This mistake was certainly not the result of their having little experience of seeing.

But how are we to respond to the other difficulties? By saying that, in fact, a man whose eyes are used to seeing sees objects more clearly than either a man-born-blind who has just had his cataracts removed or a child, whose organs are foolish and raw. Look, Madame, at all the evidence given by Monsieur l'abbé de Condillac at the end of his *Essay on the Origin of Human Knowledge*,[50] where he proposes an opposite reading of the experiments performed by Cheselden and reported by Monsieur de Voltaire. The effects of light on an eye feeling it for the first time and the conditions required in the humour of the eye, the cornea, the crystalline lens, etc. are set out with great clarity and persuasiveness there, and they make it impossible to doubt that vision occurs only very imperfectly in an infant who opens his eyes for the first time, or in a blind man who has just undergone an operation.

We must therefore agree that we must be able to grasp an infinite number of things in objects, which neither the infant nor the man-born-blind can grasp, although objects are painted inside their eyes just as they are in ours; that it is not enough for objects to make an impression on us, we must also be attentive to the impressions they make; that, as a result, we cannot see anything the first time we open our eyes; that in the first moments of vision, we can only see a multitude of blurred sensations that only become clear over time and as a result of our habitually reflecting on what is happening inside us; that it is experience alone that teaches us to compare sensations with what occasions them; that our sensations do not essentially resemble objects in any way; and that it is up to experience to teach us about the analogy between them, which seems to be purely conventional. In a word, it is impossible to doubt that touch is most useful in giving the eye a precise sense of the manner in which the object conforms to the representation of it that the eye receives, and I think that if everything did not occur in nature according to infinitely general laws, if, for example, certain hard pointed objects did not hurt to the touch and others did not provoke feelings of pleasure, we would die without having had a hundred millionth of the experiences necessary for the conservation of our bodies and for our well-being.

However, I simply do not think that the eye cannot teach itself or, if I may put it like this, give itself experience. In order to be sure of the existence and shape of the objects we touch, we do not need to be able to see them. Why then would we need to touch objects in order to be sure we could see them? I am aware of all the benefits of touch and I did not disguise them when I was discussing Saunderson or the blind man of Puiseaux; that, however, was not one I recognized. It is easy to conceive that we are able to make better and more efficient use of one sense if another one lends its support, but it is not at all easy to conceive that the senses are essentially dependent on each other for their functioning. There are certainly qualities in bodies that we would never perceive without touch; it is touch that informs us of certain features that are invisible to the eyes and which can only be seen once touch has pointed them out, but this assistance is mutual, and in those people whose sight is more acute than their touch, it is the former that tells the latter of the existence and features of objects that are so small as to escape its grasp. If a piece of paper or some other smooth, thin and flexible substance were placed between your thumb and index finger without you knowing it, only your eye could tell you that your fingers were not in direct contact with each other. I shall observe in passing that it would be infinitely more difficult to deceive a blind man in such a fashion than someone who is used to seeing.

A lively and spirited eye would no doubt find it hard to be sure that external objects were not part of itself, that it was sometimes close to them and sometimes far away, that they had a shape, that some were larger than others, that they had depth, etc., but I have no doubt at all that it would eventually see them and would be able to see them clearly enough to be able to distinguish, at least roughly, their outlines. To deny this would be to lose sight of the aim of the organs; it would be to forget the principal phenomena of vision, to pretend to oneself that no painter is talented enough to come close to the beauty and accuracy of the miniatures that are painted inside our eyes, that there is nothing more precise than the resemblance between the representation and the object represented, that the canvas of this painting is not that small, that the shapes are not blurred, that they are about half an inch square in size and that there would be nothing so difficult as explaining how touch could manage to teach the eye to see, were it absolutely impossible for the eye to see without the assistance of touch.

But I shall not rely on simple assumptions and I shall ask whether it is touch that teaches the eye to see colours? I don't think we can accord tact such an extraordinary privilege, and thus it follows that if we show a blind man who has just acquired the sense of sight a black cube and a red sphere on a large white background, it will not take him long to see the edges of the shapes.

It will take as long as it takes, one might argue, for the eye's humours to settle properly, for the cornea to acquire the necessary convex shape, for the pupil to be able to dilate and contract as it should, for the retina's filaments to be neither too sensitive nor too insensitive to the effect of the light, for the crystalline lens to perform the forward and backward movements we suspect it makes, for the muscles to perform their functions properly, for the optic nerves to become accustomed to transmitting sensation, for the whole eyeball to arrange itself in the necessary manner and for all the parts that make up the eyeball to work together to execute the miniature of which we make such good use; that's how long it will take before the eye is able to give itself experience. I confess that however simple a picture I show the man-born-blind, he will only be able to distinguish its parts once his eyes have fulfilled all the preceding conditions, but that may only take an instant, and it would not be difficult to apply the argument that has just been put to me to a fairly complex mechanism such as a watch, and prove by listing all the movements that occur in the barrel, the fusee, the wheels, the pallets, the balance, etc. that it would take two weeks for the second hand to move. If the reply to that is that those movements happen simultaneously, I shall reply that the same may be true of the ones that occur in the eye when it opens for the first time and of the judgements that take place as a result. Whatever you make of the conditions that are necessary for the eye to be able to see, you must agree that it is not touch that creates them, that the eye acquires them by itself and that as a result, it will succeed in distinguishing the shapes that are painted inside it without the assistance of another sense.

But I hear you say once again, when will it be able to do so? Perhaps more quickly than you think. When we went to the King's Garden together, do you remember, Madame, seeing the concave mirror, and how frightened you were when you saw the tip of a sword coming towards you at the same speed as that at which the tip of the one you had in your hand was moving towards the surface of the mirror? And yet you are used to relating objects in mirrors to a space beyond them. Experience is thus neither as necessary nor as infallible as we think when it comes to perceiving objects or their images in the right places. Even your parrot proves my point. The first time he saw himself in a mirror, he went up close to it with his beak, and when he did not encounter his brother who was, in fact, himself, he walked round the back of the glass. I don't want to make too much of the parrot's evidence, but as an animal, preconceived ideas can have no part in its experience.

However, if you were to tell me that a man-born-blind would not be able to see anything for two months, I should not be surprised. I should simply conclude that the organ needs experience and not that it needs touch for that experience. I should merely have a clearer understanding of the importance of letting a blind man who will be the object of these observations rest in the dark, of allowing his eyes to exercise, which they can do much more comfortably in darkness than in light, and of putting him in a kind of dusk for the experiments or at least in a place where it is possible for him to choose to have more or less light. It would make me all the more inclined to agree that these kinds of experiments are always very difficult and very uncertain, and that the quickest way of doing them, though seemingly the longest, is to equip the subject with philosophical training sufficient to enable him to compare the two conditions he has known and to acquaint us with the difference between the state of a blind person and that of one who can see. I say it again, how precise can one expect someone to be if they are not used to thinking and self-examination, and if they, like Cheselden's blind man, are so unaware of the benefits of sight that they are ignorant of their misfortune and cannot imagine how the loss of that sense impairs their pleasures? Saunderson, whom we cannot refuse the title of philosopher, was certainly not indifferent to his loss, and I very much doubt whether he would have been of the opinion of the author of the excellent *Treatise on Systems*. I rather suspect the latter philosopher of having indulged in a system himself when he says that, 'if man's life had been nothing other an uninterrupted sensation of pleasure or pain, either happy with no idea of unhappiness, or unhappy with no idea of happiness, he would have known only pleasure or suffering; and as if that were his very nature, he would never have looked around to see whether some being was keeping a protective watch over him or plotting to do him harm. It is the shift from one state to the other which made him think, etc.'[51]

Madame, do you think it was by proceeding from one clear idea to another (for that is the author's way of philosophizing and the right one) that he arrived at such a conclusion? Happiness and unhappiness are not like darkness and light; the one does not consist in the pure and simple deprivation of the other. We might perhaps have said that happiness was no less essential to us than existence and thought, had we enjoyed it without interruption, but I cannot say the same of unhappiness. It would have been perfectly natural to think of it as an enforced condition, to feel oneself to be innocent yet believe oneself to be guilty, and blame or excuse nature, which is what we do.

Does Monsieur l'abbé de Condillac think a child only cries when he is in pain because he has not been in pain without respite since he was born? If he were to reply that 'existing and suffering would be one and the same for someone who had always been suffering, and he would be unable to imagine that his pain could come to an end without his existence coming to an end too,' I should reply in turn that, though the man who had constantly been unhappy would perhaps not have said, 'What have I done to deserve this pain?', what would have prevented him from asking, 'What I have done to exist?'? Moreover, I see no reason why he wouldn't have had two synonyms, *I exist* and *I suffer*, one for prose and one for poetry, just as we have two expressions, *I live* and *I breathe*. However, you will observe better than I, Madame, that this part of Monsieur l'abbé de Condillac is very beautifully written, and I rather fear you will say, as you compare my criticism with his observations, that you would still rather an error by Montaigne than a truth by Charron.[52]

You're digressing again, I hear you say. Yes, Madame, it is the very nature of our treatise. Now, here is my opinion on the two previous questions. I think that the first time the blind man's eyes receive light, he will see nothing at all. His eye will need some time to give itself experience, but it will do so on its own and without the help of touch, and it will succeed not only in seeing colours but also in making out the rough edges of objects. Now let us see whether, supposing he acquires this ability in a very short space of time or gains it by exercising his eyes in the darkness, as he had been told to do by those who carefully confined him to it for some time after the operation and before the experiments, let us see, I say, whether he would recognize by his sight the bodies he had touched, and whether he would be able to give them the appropriate names. This is the last question I have to answer.

In order to do so in a manner that will please you, since you are fond of method, I shall distinguish between several kinds of persons on whom the experiments may be carried out. If they are common people with no education or knowledge and who have not been trained for it, I think that, were the operation to remove the defect completely from the eye and the eye to be healthy, the objects would be painted very clearly inside it, but that such people who are unused to any kind of rational thought, not knowing what is meant by sensation or idea and unable to compare the representations they have gained from touch with those they have gained from their eyes, would declare, 'That's the circle, that's the square', without there being any basis for their judgement. Alternatively, they may even naively agree that they could perceive nothing in the objects now present to their sight that resembled those they were used to touching.

There are other people who, by comparing the shapes they would perceive to the bodies whose shapes used to impress themselves on their hands, and by mentally applying their sense of touch to those bodies at a distance, would say of one that it was a square and the other that it was a circle, but without knowing why, because the comparison between the ideas gained by touch and those received by sight would not occur in them clearly enough for them to be certain of the truth of their judgment.

I shall turn now, Madame, without digressing, to a metaphysician on whom one might try the experiment. I have no doubt that from the very first moment he saw them clearly, he would, by contrast, think about the shapes as if he had been able to see them all his life, and that having compared the ideas that came to him by his eyes with those he gained by his touch, he would say, with the same assurance as you and I, that, 'I should be tempted to believe that this body is the one I have always called circle and this the one I have always called square, but I shall refrain from saying so. Who says that were I to approach them, they wouldn't disappear from beneath my hands? How do I know whether the objects I can see are destined also to be the objects of my touch? I do not know whether what is visible is also palpable. However, even if I were not uncertain of this and took the people around me at their word when they say that what I can see really is what I touched, I should not be any better off. Those objects could easily change in my hands and transmit sensations by my tact that are the very opposite of those I have sensed by my sight. Gentlemen, he would add, this body seems to me to be the square and this the circle, but I cannot know for certain that they feel the same as they look.'

If we replaced the metaphysician by a geometer, Locke by Saunderson, he would also say that, were he to believe his eyes, of the two figures he could see, this is the one he would call a square, and this the circle, 'for I can see,' he would add, 'that the first one is the only one that would allow me to arrange threads and position large-headed pins in such a way as to mark out the corners of a square, and the second one is the only one that I can inscribe or circumscribe with the threads necessary for the demonstration of the properties of a circle. So, that's the circle, and that's the square! However,' he would have continued, following Locke, 'perhaps when I come to apply my hands to the shapes, one will change into the other such that the same shape could serve to demonstrate the properties of a circle to blind people and to those who can see, the properties of a square. Perhaps I should see a square and at the same time, feel a circle. No,' he would continue, 'I am wrong. Those people who witnessed my demonstration of the properties of the circle and the square did not have their hands on my abacus, and they couldn't touch the threads I had tied to make the outlines of my shapes; yet they could understand me. Therefore, they were not seeing a square when I was feeling a circle, otherwise we would never have understood each other for I should have been drawing one shape and demonstrating the properties of another, giving them a straight line instead of a curve, and a curve instead of a straight line. Yet since they all understood me, must everyone therefore see in the same way? I therefore see a square when they see a square and a circle when they see a circle. So that's what I have always called a square, and that's what I have always called a circle.'

I have substituted circle for sphere and square for cube, because it very much appears that we can only judge distance by experience, and as a result, someone using his eyes for the first time will only see surfaces and not understand projection, which consists in some of its points of a body seeming to be closer to us than others.

Yet even if the man-born-blind were able to judge of the projection and solidity of bodies from the very first moments of clear vision and tell the difference not only between the circle and the square but also between the sphere and the cube, I nonetheless do not believe he would be able to do the same for more composite objects. It would very much seem that Monsieur de Réaumur's girl-born-blind could tell colours apart, but I bet you thirty to one she guessed the sphere and the cube, and I am certain that, short of some revelation, she was unable to recognize her gloves, dressing gown and slippers. These objects are laden with so many modifications, and their overall shape bears so little relationship to the parts of the body they are designed to adorn or cover, that Saunderson would have found it a hundred times more difficult to work out what his square bonnet was for than it would be for Monsieur d'Alembert or Monsieur Clairaut to work out what his tables were for.[53]

Saunderson would not have failed to suppose there to be a geometrical relationship between things and their use and he would therefore have realized by means of two or three analogies that his skullcap was made for his head, since its shape has nothing arbitrary about it to mislead him. But what would he have thought of the corners and the tassel of his mortar board? 'What's the point of the tassel? And why four corners and not six?' he would have wondered. And those two features, which are a decorative matter to us, would have been the source of a whole host of absurdities to him or, rather, the opportunity for an excellent satire on what we call good taste.

All things seriously considered, we must confess that between someone who has always been able to see but who doesn't know what an object is for, and someone who knows what an object is for but has never been able to see, the latter does not have the advantage. However, do you believe, Madame, that, were you shown a headdress for the first time today, you could manage to work out that it is a dressing to go on your head? Yet if it is that much more difficult for a man-born-blind who can see for the first time to judge correctly what an object is because of the many forms it can take, what would prevent him from thinking that an observer who was fully clothed from head to toe and sitting motionless in an armchair in front of him was not a piece of furniture or a machine, and that a tree with its branches and leaves waving in the wind was not a self-moving, animate and thinking being? Madame, how many things our senses suggest to us, and if we didn't have eyes, how difficult we would find it to suppose that a block of marble could not think and feel!

So it is obvious that it is only with respect to the circle and the square that Saunderson would have been sure his judgement was not wrong, and that there are cases in which the reasoning and experience of others can clarify how sight relates to touch, and teach the sense of sight that what is so for the eye is also so for the hand.

Yet it would nonetheless be essential in any attempt to demonstrate some eternally true proposition, as they are called, to test such a demonstration by performing it in the absence of sensible evidence because, Madame, you will see that were someone to set about proving to you that two parallel lines should be drawn on a plane as two convergent lines because that is how two paths look, he would be forgetting that the proposition is as true for a blind man as it is for him.

And the previous supposition regarding the man-born-blind suggests two more: one about a man who had been able to see since birth but had no sense of touch, and the other about a man whose senses of sight and touch constantly contradicted each other. It might be asked of the first man whether, were he accorded the sense he lacked and deprived of the sense of sight by a blindfold, he would be able to recognize the bodies by his touch. It is obvious that geometry, were he to have any knowledge of it, would provide him with an infallible way of discovering whether or not his senses contradicted each other. He would have only to pick up the cube or the sphere, demonstrate some of its properties to others and declare, provided they could understand him, that they were seeing as a cube what he was feeling as one, and that it was therefore the cube he was holding. As for the man who had no knowledge of this science, I think he would find it no easier to distinguish the cube and the sphere by his touch than Mr Molyneux's blind man would by his sight.

With respect to the man whose sensations of sight and

touch were in constant contradiction, I don't know what he would think of shapes, order, symmetry, beauty, ugliness, etc. It would very much appear that he would know as much about them as we do about the size and duration of animal life in relation to real space and time. He would make the general declaration that a body has a shape, but he would necessarily be inclined to think that it is neither the one he sees nor the one he feels. Such a man could easily be discontented with his senses, but his senses could neither be contented nor discontented with their objects. If he were tempted to accuse one of them of lying, I think it would be his sense of touch. A hundred details would incline him to think that an object changes shape when his hands act on it rather than when it acts on his eyes. Yet such preconceptions would mean that the different degrees of hardness and softness that he could observe in bodies would trouble him.

Yet if our senses do not contradict each other over shapes, does this mean that shapes are any better known to us? How do we know that our senses are not deceiving us? And yet we make judgements nonetheless. Alas! Madame, once we have weighed human knowledge in Montaigne's scales, we are not far from adopting his motto.[54] For what do we know? What matter is? Absolutely not. What mind and thought are? Even less so. What movement, space and duration are? Not at all. Geometrical truths? Ask any honest mathematician and he will tell you that his propositions are all identical, and that all those tomes devoted to the circle, for example, can be reduced to the same statement which they make in a hundred, thousand different ways, namely that it is a shape in which all the lines leading from the centre to the circumference are equal. We know therefore almost nothing, and yet how many works there are whose authors have all claimed to know something. I cannot imagine why people do not tire of reading and yet learning nothing, unless it is for the same reason that I have had the honour of conversing with you for two hours without either boring myself or telling you anything. I am, with the deepest respect,

MADAME,

Your most humble and most obedient servant,

***

Index[55]

Notes

1 'They can, but they don't seem to be able to'. The line is adapted from Virgil; see above, pp. 24–6.
2 The real place of publication was Paris.
3 René Antoine Ferchault, Seigneur de Réaumur et de La Bermondière (1683–1757), member of the Académie Royale des Sciences [Royal Academy of the Sciences] since 1708 and elected its Director on eleven occasions. He was most famous for his six-volume study of insects, *Mémoires pour servir à l'histoire des insectes* [Memoirs for Use in the Study of Insects], 6 volumes (Paris: Imprimerie Royale, 1734–42).
4 According to Rousseau's *Confessions*, this remark may have been what triggered Diderot's arrest and imprisonment (Jean-Jacques Rousseau, *Confessions*, Angela Scholar (trans.), Patrick Coleman (ed., intro. and notes) (Oxford: Oxford World's Classics, 2008), p. 338).
5 Joseph Hillmer (born c. 1720), Prussian oculist; see above pp. 127–9.
6 She may be a relation of the Simoneau who was one the engravers of Réaumur's *Mémoires*.
7 The King's Garden [Jardin du Roi], directed by Georges Leclerc, comte de Buffon (1707–1788) since 1739.
8 There is some evidence for his real-life existence, see above pp. 38–41.
9 René Descartes, *Dioptrics* (1637). The figure reproduced in the *Letter* is taken from an eighteenth-century edition and differs in significant ways from the original; see above pp. 60, 72.
10 René Hérault, Seigneur de Fontaine-l'Abbé et de Vaucresson (1691–1740), Lieutenant General of the Paris Police (1725–1739).
11 This is a reversal of Montaigne's description of a good marriage as one between a blind wife and a deaf husband (*Essays*, in *The Complete Works: Essays, Travel Journal, Letters*, Donald M. Frame (trans.), Stuart Hampshire (intro.) (London: Everyman, 2003), p. 804).
12 Diogenes was a Greek Cynical philosopher, known for his lewd and provocative behaviour that challenged social customs.
13 For a history of this term, see Daniel Heller-Roazen, *The Inner Touch* (Cambridge, MA: MIT Press, 2007).
14 Descartes located the soul in the pineal gland, see *The Passions of the Soul* (1649), in *The Philosophical Writings of Descartes*, vol. 1.
15 For a discussion of medical theories of the nerves and brain, see Ann Thomson, *Bodies of Thought: Science, Religion, and the Soul in the Early Enlightenment* (Oxford: Oxford University Press, 2008), pp. 175–215.

16 For a history of this term, see Peter Dear, 'The Meanings of Experience', in *The Cambridge History of Science*, David C. Lindberg and Ronald L. Numbers (eds), 7 volumes (Cambridge: Cambridge University Press, 2003), vol. 3, pp. 106–31, especially the section entitled 'Event Experiments and 'Physico-Mathematics', pp. 124–30.

17 Pythagoras, Greek mathematician and mystical philosopher.

18 The Index reveals the English geometer to be Joseph Raphson (died 1712?); the phrase is to be found in Latin in the final lines of his work, *Analysis æquationum universalis, seu, Ad æquationes algebraicas resolvendas methodus generalis, & expedita, ex nova infinitarum serierum methodo, deducta ac demonstrata. Editio secunda cum appendice; cui annexum est, De spatio reali, seu entre infinito conamen mathematico-metaphysicum* (London: Typis T. Braddyll, prostant venales apud Johannem Taylor, 1697).

19 Nicholas Saunderson (1682–1739), mathematician, holder of the Lucasian Chair of Mathematics at the University of Cambridge (1711–1739), and author of the posthumously published *The Elements of Algebra, in Ten Books: by Nicholas Saunderson LL.D. Late Lucasian Professor of the mathematics in the University of Cambridge, and Fellow of the Royal Society. To which is prefixed, an account of the author's life and character, collected from his oldest and most intimate acquaintances*, 2 volumes (Cambridge: Printed at the University-Press: and sold by Mrs. Saunderson at Cambridge, by John Whiston bookseller at Boyle's Head in Fleet Street London, and Thomas Hammond in York, 1740).

20 There is no evidence for Saunderson's literary achievements; is the text is hinting that the Saunderson of the *Letter* is, at least in part, a literary creation?

21 Much of what follows is taken from John Colson, 'Saunderson's Palpable Arithmetic Decyphered', in Saunderson, *Elements*, vol. 1, pp. xx–xxvi.

22 This appears to be a mistake and should read 'right' not 'left'. Given Diderot's fondness for reversals and puzzles, it is not impossible that the mistake is deliberate, designed perhaps to test the limits of the reader's concentration.

23 See Saunderson, *Elements*, vol. 1, p. xxiv.

24 See Saunderson, *Elements*, vol. 1, p. xxiv.

25 See Saunderson, *Elements*, vol. 1, p. xxiv.

26 See Saunderson, *Elements*, vol. 1, p. xxiv.

27 See note 18.

28 See Saunderson, *Elements*, vol. 1, p. iv.

29 The Index reveals 'Monsieur de M . . .' to be Pierre Carlet de Chamblain de Marivaux (1688–1763), journalist, novelist and

playwright. A number of the ideas in the preceding section echo his 'Du Style' [On Style]. See *Le Cabinet du philosophe* (1734) in *Journaux et œuvres diverses* (Paris: Garnier, 1969), pp. 380–88.

30 Tacitus, Roman historian, known for his difficult Latin.

31 George Berkeley, *Three Dialogues between Hylas and Philonous* (London: printed by G. James for Henry Clements, 1713); a French translation, *Dialogues entre Hylas et Philonous*, by the mathematician and Encyclopedist, Jean Paul Gua de Malves (1713–1785), was published in Amsterdam in 1744.

32 Etienne Bonnot de Condillac, *Essay on the Origin of Human Knowledge* [1746], Hans Aarsleff (trans.) (Cambridge: Cambridge University Press, 2001).

33 This is a close quotation of the first paragraph of the first chapter of Condillac's *Essay*, which reads 'Whether we raise ourselves, metaphorically speaking, into the heavens or descend into the abyss, we do not go beyond ourselves; and we never perceive anything but our own thought' (p. 11). The omission of the qualification, 'metaphorically speaking', is key to enabling the comparison with Berkeley.

34 It had appeared earlier in 1749.

35 See Saunderson, 'Memoirs', in *Elements*, vol. 1, p. xii.

36 These are all famous blind men of antiquity, listed in Saunderson, 'Memoirs', in *Elements*, vol. 1, pp. ix–x.

37 Gervaise Holmes seems to have been Saunderson's vicar, see Saunderson, 'Memoirs', in *Elements*, vol. 1, p. xix.

38 References to this 'Indian' philosophy can be found in a number of French and English writers of the period; see Fontenelle, 'Premier Soir' [First Evening], *Entretiens sur la pluralité des mondes* [Conversations on the Plurality of Worlds] (1686); Locke, *Essay Concerning Human Understanding* (1690), book 2, chapter 13, paragraph 9, and chapter 23, paragraph 2; Maillet, *Telliamed, ou, entretiens d'un philosophe indien avec un missionnaire français sur la diminution de la mer* [Telliamed, or Conversations between an Indian Philosopher and a French Missionary on the Diminution of the Sea] (c. 1692–1708, publ. 1748); Shaftesbury, *The Moralists* (1711), Part 1, section 2; Diderot, *De la suffisance de la religion naturelle* [On the Sufficiency of Natural Religion] (1746), paragraph 22.

39 These three names had been associated with each other since the publication in 1717 of parts of the correspondence between Leibniz and Clarke, in which the latter defended Newton's ideas, notably those on the attributes of God, against Leibniz's criticisms, see *The Leibniz-Clarke Correspondence*, H. G. Alexander (ed.) (Manchester: Manchester University Press, 1956).

40 Much of what follows echoes Lucretius, *De Rerum natura* [On the Nature of the Universe], book 4, lines 835–860 and book 2, lines 1060–70.
41 His question echoes that asked by the disciples to Jesus, see John 9.2.
42 See Saunderson, 'Memoirs', in *Elements*, vol. 1, p. xix.
43 The title is close to that of the 'Memoirs of the Life and Character of Dr. Nicholas Saunderson', but no such work has been found.
44 See Saunderson, 'Memoirs', in *Elements*, vol. 1, p. xii.
45 Democritus, Greek atomist philosopher. The story about him gouging out his own eyes is reported in, for example, Aulus Gellius, *Noctes Atticæ* [Attic Nights], book 10, chapter 17.
46 See Locke, *Essay*, book 2, chapter 9, paragraph 8.
47 Ibid.
48 Condillac's discussion of Molyneux's Problem is to be found in the *Essay*, pp. 100–10.
49 It had appeared in 1738.
50 They are to be found at the end of the first part of Condillac's *Essay*.
51 See Condillac, *Œuvres philosophiques*, Georges Le Roy (ed.), 3 volumes (Paris: Presses Universitaires de France, 1947), vol. 1, p. 134.
52 This is an echo of Pascal's comparison between the two writers (*Pensées and Other Writings*, Honor Levi (trans.), Anthony Levi (intro. and notes) (Oxford: Oxford World's Classics, 2008), p. 139). This edition uses the Sellier classification and gives the fragment as number 644.
53 Jean Le Rond d'Alembert (1717–1783), mathematician and co-editor with Diderot of the *Encyclopédie*; Alexis Claude Clairaut (1713–1765), mathematician.
54 Montaigne's motto was 'Que sçays-je?' [What do I know?] inscribed over a pair of scales, see Montaigne, *Essays*, p. 477.
55 The Index is Diderot's.

Appendix Two

François de La Mothe Le Vayer, 'Of a Man-Born-Blind' (1653)

Note on the Translation

This is the first English translation and the first modern edition of François de La Mothe Le Vayer's 'D'un Aveugle-nay', which first appeared in his *Suite de petits traités en forme de lettres, écrites à diverses personnes studieuses*, 2 volumes (Paris: A. Courbé, 1653).

The marginal notes are La Mothe Le Vayer's. The endnotes are mine and have been kept to a minimum. I have provided translations of the Greek, Latin and Spanish in square brackets in the text only in those cases where the preceding or following sentence of the original is not itself a translation. I am grateful to Emma Herdman for her help with the Greek.

Sir,

When Galen wished to describe the marvels of the eye and the importance of sight, he protested that he was doing so at the express command of a Divinity. He apologized for going against the tastes of the doctors of his time by making use of geometrical demonstrations and said those were the orders of the God who prescribed him the work.* Had this great interpreter of nature's most secret mysteries not wished to speak of the genius that had forced him into such a fine contemplation, every man since Socrates having a genius of his own,

Lib. 10, *de usu partium*, c.12, 13 &14.

> . . . *Sua cuique Deus fit dira cupido*
> [Each person's ruling passion is his God]

Virgil.

I should have found his words rather harsh, particularly for a man of his profession, and the most devoted followers of his doctrine would perhaps find it quite difficult to defend his sincerity and even to relate this passage to many others in his work. Whatever the case, since I wish only to talk to you of the impairment and the defects of the eye or, rather, of the total deprivation of sight, I have no need to take God as my guarantor as he did, and it will be enough for me to say that in answer to your curiosity about the entertainments I may be enjoying in Poitiers, I wish to report to you the conversation I had with a man-born-blind whom I have been shown while here.

Indeed I could hardly choose a subject more suitable for your attention, since opposites are understood in relation to each other, and privations in relation to habits. We can only properly understand darkness in relation to light, and blindness in relation to the functioning of the eye and the excellence of sight. Now, you know that sight is the noblest of the senses and the eye the most important part of the human body, in which it occupies, Aristotle says, the same place as that of reason in the soul of which it is the noblest part, ωσπερ εν σωματι οψις εν ψυχη νους.[1] If its rank could be challenged, it would doubtless be by hearing, which is truly not for reasons without foundation called the sense of the disciplines and even that of faith, and which since the majority of the sciences are achromatic, as the Scholastics put it, and reliant on the voice to be understood, is in this respect doubtless worthy of much praise. However, we must admit that if we compare these two senses, sight must always win on many counts. It is not without good reason that a visual witness is worth ten of those who report only what they have heard said, *plus valet oculatus testis unus, quam auriti decem* [one eye witness is worth ten ear witnesses].[2] Words, which pass through the ivory entrance hall that is symbolized by the teeth, are capable of much greater deception than objects that come to us by way of the cornea or through the medium of the eye's corneal membrane, according to Servius's interpretation.[3] Moreover, generally speaking, sight imprints things much more powerfully in our souls than hearing does:

> *Segnius irritant animos demissa per aurem,*
> *Quam que sunt oculis subjecta fidelibus.*

Horat., *de arte poetica.*

This is the basis for the fine mythological story that has come down to us from Lucian, relating what the Ancients said about the Sirens and the Gorgons.[4] The former could not instantly attract men because they needed time to be understood and so some men managed to escape them. But the effect of the Gorgons, who acted by means of sight alone and had no recourse to hearing, was immediate and so swift that no one ever managed to resist them. There are even some sciences like astronomy to which, it can be claimed, the eyes have made a far greater contribution than the other senses. The Hebrews call those with the gift of prophesy nothing other than seers, though the reference is principally to the mind. And I recall that Plato maintains in his *Timaeus* that philosophy, the greatest of all the gifts (he says) that the gods wished to give men, was communicated to us by sight.[5] That is why I am not so surprised by another of Galen's thoughts about the location of our eyes. Many people have been content to follow Macrobius and say that all the senses are found in the head, which is where reason is to be found because the senses must be subservient to reason. But Galen thinks sight is so important that he claims the brain, which he understands to be the location of reason, is only in the head because that is where the eyes are, and that they have to be there because it is the most elevated place in the body. He does, however, accept that the other senses are in the head because that is where the brain is. This is truly to accord a marvellous superiority to sight. And certainly the way sight operates instantaneously on so many different things does indeed reveal that it is wholly celestial.

Lib. 7. *Saturn*, cap. 14.

Lib. 8. *De usu part.*, cap. 5.

The other four senses have obvious relations to the other elements and this leaves sight whose relationship to the heavens is the closest and highest of all. It is by means of this fifth sense that man alone can enjoy the delights of painting and the other rare and subtle qualities of the arts. And it seems to me that it is the eyes alone that led the Greeks to call the human face, προσωοπον, because, Aristotle says, πρόσωσθευ οπωπε, man is, of all the animals, the only one that can look straight ahead. These same Greeks conferred no small prerogative on sight over the other senses, whose other organs are, however, no less visible and recognisable on the human face than those of sight.

3. *De part. ani.*, c. 1.

But I haven't noticed how long this prologue has become; it may perhaps be even longer than the main piece. So, to return to the blind man about whom I proposed to talk to you and with whom I had a conversation, his name is Dreux la Vallée. He is a gentleman of one of the good houses of Poitiers who, despite his misfortune, nonetheless attended the Colleges and advanced far enough in his studies to be able publicly to dispute philosophical theses. He initially told me he was unsure whether he had been born with a total lack of sight, since he was told by his parents that they had only become aware of his *blindness* when he was nine or ten months old, but he was certain he had no memory of ever having seen anything. I considered his vision to be quite clear and asked him whether, when he was in the light and in the sunlight in particular, he could not tell that the air was brighter than it was inside or when it was dark. To begin with he said no, but once I took him over to the window and made him first turn to face the light and then turn his back on it, he recognized that he could make out some difference, which he had until then always thought came from some thickening of the air, which he could feel when he approached a wall or some other solid object, rather than from the light. Indeed you will notice that he can walk around his room without bumping into anything, which is something we are unable to do when we are in the dark, and he would be able to walk through the town with no need of a guide, he said, if the only thing he had to fear was bumping into walls. Because he protests that he cannot see anything, he attributes his ability to a kind of instinct, as he calls it, and to a pre-notion that nature gives him by means of the condensation of the air, which he can somehow feel when he comes close to a physical mass that makes it rebound. I think it is simply an effect of the light acting on his eyes regardless of their impairment, just as it does on our eyes when we close them. Having out eyes shut does not prevent us from being able to tell the difference between day and night, or from seeing a candle in the dark. Nor is his *blindness* such that he cannot perceive the darkness of a body that makes the air less light and informs him almost imperceptibly that his path would be blocked if he tried to proceed any further.

As for colours, he knows them only through what he has been taught about them in physics lessons. He knows that there are some that are true just as there are others that are merely apparent, and that between black and white there are five medium colours as well an infinity of others that depend on how much or how little of the first two they contain. Although he talks in a different way to that in which blind people usually talk about colours, he nonetheless assures us that he is unable to see any of them, and even that he is unable to imagine what they could in fact be.

I asked him whether he had any idea of the sun or the moon and the great multitude of stars that rotate with the firmament above our heads. He replied that he had some knowledge of the movements of the heavens, which he had acquired by feeling the globe he had been given to touch by the people who had taught him some astronomy. In fact, he is not unaware of the series of the sun's positions on the obliquity of the zodiac, and he can understand that the distance between the polar circles and the pole is the same as that between the tropics and the equator. But despite all that, he asked us to believe that he had not the slightest conjecture of the beauty of either the great star, the marvels of which he heard so much about, or everything he was assured was visible in the heavens to anyone able to contemplate them.

You can see in all this clear proof of the philosophical axiom according to which nothing enters our minds except by way of the senses, and as a result, if one sense is lacking, the soul is necessarily deprived of much knowledge. To enlighten myself further, I asked him if, when he slept, he had ever dreamed that he was talking to his friends, and if so, whether they seemed to him to be wearing clothes, since even if his imagination were to represent them to him naked, their bodies would have to appear clothed in some colour. He recognized that his fantasy had often afforded him such illusions, but he said he never saw his friends in these conversations, which only involved words or entertainments in which no colour of any kind was present, just as in the conversation we were having he could not see us, despite his talking to us and our communicating with each other. I had asked him that question because, given the internal faculty that we call fantasy which, according to its Greek etymology, is another light that illuminates within and which perhaps made Tiberius and Cardano blind for a short while after they awoke,[6] I wished to discover whether it could provide him with some independent phantom in his naturally lacking state. But I had the common doctrine confirmed according to which that second light depends absolutely on the first; it is *lumen de lumine* [light of light] and it illuminates in colour only if colours have been revealed through the windows of the soul, which are the eyes.

'απο του φαους' Arist. 3. *De ani.* Cap. 14.

While staying here, I have also been shown another blind man whose father was a watchmaker and who has made various pieces by hand and with some skill. Someone gave Cardinal de Richelieu a special present of a miniature carriage he had made in a very dark cellar so that he would be less distracted in his work than elsewhere or so that he could share with moles not only their blindness but also their liking for life underground. However, I observed nothing more remarkable in his work than in that of the blind man who lives in the Hospital for the Blind in Paris[7] and makes cobbler's lasts and polishes them so beautifully. He is less remarkable than the first blind man in that he was not born blind and can remember having seen stars in the sky because he lost his sight when he was four years old. The word 'aveugle' [blind] comes from the Latin *aboculatus* and it is therefore the right word for him since he has lost the sight he once had, but he is not blind from birth or *cæcus ab ortu*. So it seems that if we are to speak correctly, the man-born-blind should not be called *aboculatus* nor simply 'aveugle' because he cannot lose what he never possessed. Usage nonetheless triumphs here, as it does elsewhere over such minor grammatical considerations. We know for certain that not all people who have been born blind remain so, for Tartars are born into the world with their eyes closed like dogs and only see clearly, as many writers have observed, after five days. It has also been said that the eye is the last organ to be formed by nature because it is the least necessary, which does not diminish the importance we have given it. In truth, it is said that, like some imperfect animals such as those we see in shells, the whale needs to be led by a guide because it cannot see anything. Moles have eyes, but it is thought that they are covered by a membrane that renders them useless. Antonius Diogenes asserts in *Photius* that the men of a town in Iberia can only see in the dark and can see nothing at all in the daylight.[8] And since the Issedones, who are the Scythian Arimaspoi, are one-eyed,[9] it seems that nature does not take as much care with sight as she ordinarily does with things that are absolutely necessary.

That would not offer much consolation to those who have lost their sight, but there are certainly some much stronger arguments that can make their plight seem less disastrous. How much pain and suffering are they spared by virtue of the general moral maxim that says we never wish for anything of which we are ignorant? *Ignoti nulla cupido*. Being deprived of the greatest pleasures afforded to us by the sense of sight is not, as some would claim, something that can make those who are blind from birth unhappy if that maxim is as correct as we think it is. Let us suppose nonetheless that they are to be pitied for the loss of the many pleasures that sight could afford them, but how much unpleasantness are they spared in return? And are we not obliged to admit, if we consider this point properly, that they are better off since they gain more than they lose in their blindness? For it cannot be said that blindness is a bad thing in itself and considered on its own, unless we wish to claim that we spend half or nearly half our lives in misery because we have our eyes closed. This is not the case at all and, if we pay attention, we realize that we often close them in order better to taste the pleasures of the other senses and make our soul more receptive, as it always is when it is less distracted. In fact, when the poet wanted to represent Dido in her greatest moment of happiness, he deprived her of light and put her deep inside a dark cave:

> *Speluncam Dido, dux et Trojanus eandem Deveniunt.*
> [Dido and the Trojan both came to this cave.][10]

To judge a tune or really appreciate the taste of fine wine, nature herself leads us to close our eyes. And darkness is sometimes so satisfying that we seek it out even in the most sacred things, for the dark air of temples increases our faith and the heavens never appear brighter to our souls than when we are in a dark place or when it is night and we cannot see anything around us.

How many stories refer to remarkable blind men such as Appius Claudius, who saw important matters more clearly than the most clear-sighted of his time? And is it not said of Democritus that he deliberately deprived himself of his physical eyes so as to improve his spiritual ones and improve their contemplative powers, unless he did so, as others claim, to avoid suffering the sight of evil men who prospered no less in his time than they have done since. Homer's blindness did not stop him from making us see things that were so beautiful that more than two thousand years later, everyone still admires them. And Tiresias, who saw so clearly into the future that he was taken to be the greatest of the Gentile prophets, was no less blind than Homer, although, as Cicero observes, poets do not represent 5. *Tus. qu.* him lamenting his fate as they do Polyphemus who, in his primitive state, thought he had lost everything when he lost his sight. In truth, they would have been quite wrong to give such a crude man's feelings to a man who they say received so many gracious gifts from Jupiter, especially since the blind are not like the deaf and the dumb, who can never become, so Aristotle says, judicious and wise like the Lib. *De sensibi.* former. c. 1. Prudence is so close to blindness that many people who wish to appear prudent pretend to suffer from short sight. This is something of which the Spanish are often accused since they start wearing *antojos* [spectacles] earlier than most people, or at least they do so *por gravedad* [out of seriousness], as they say, which is another quality they seek.

We can go further, however, and claim that sight is often the cause of more misery than blindness. Ovid was banished for having seen too much, and many others since have found themselves in situations of great misfortune for the same reason. Ovid's Medea fears that her eyes will be criminal:

> *. . . oculosque videndo Conscelero*
> [. . . profane my eyes at the sight of it] Lib. 7. *Metam.*

We are not only fascinated by what we see but we are also the objects of others' fascinated gazes. There are some powerful monarchs on earth who are so feeble-minded that they punish anyone who looks at them and, if Acosta is to be believed, it was a crime punishable by death for a member of the lower classes to look at the king of Mexico.[11] How many people can repeat the words of that unfortunate lover: *ut vidi, ut perii* [I saw her and I was lost]?[12] And who can boast of ever having come home from town without that part of us that allows us to see having been assaulted, often in many different ways. So it is no great surprise that the Hebrew wise man exclaimed in his book, Ecclesiasticus, *nequius oculo quid creatum est!* ['A wicked eye is an evil thing!].[13]

In truth, it cannot be denied that the absence of sight can sometimes be a disadvantage. It is because of it that some have been forbidden to wear the crown to which they might otherwise have pretended. Manilus Torquatus is praised for having turned down the role of consul on account of his eyes, refusing it on the grounds that someone who sees through someone else's eyes cannot, without being presumptuous, accept a responsibility that places the life and goods of an infinite number of people in his hands and at his discretion.[14] In short, unless we succumb to mental blindness, we shall never underestimate the disadvantages of physical blindness. But on the other hand, you will see that greater ones are not avoided by being able to see, and you will have to admit that blindness has its advantages and privileges, some of which are even greater than those we have observed so far, not least that we step into the gutter for the blind, as we do for the greatest noblemen. In conclusion, allow me this little mockery in favour of the former, and let me say that if Aristotle's text is correct and that for pigs, losing an eye means losing their life, it may be said that we would be more like pigs than reasonable men if we could not live without eyes.[15]

Notes

1 Aristotle, *Nicomachean Ethics*, book 1, chapter 6, lines 1096b28–30.

2 Plautus, *Truculentus*, lines 489–90.

3 Servius, *Commentary on Virgil's Æneid*, book 6, line 893.

4 Lucian, *De Domo* [The Hall], in *The Works of Lucian*, A. M. Harmon (trans.), 8 volumes (London: William Heinemann; New York: Macmillan, 1913), vol. 1, pp. 195–6.

5 Plato, *Timaeus*, 47a–c.

6 Suetonius, *The Lives of the Cæsars*, 3: 68.2; Girolamo Cardano said of his father that he could see in the dark (*De Vita propria* [The Book of My Life], chapter 3). The reference may be

to Cardano's dreams, for which he was well known in the period, see *De Vita propria*, chapter 37. In the same chapter, Cardano claims he could always see the moon even in daylight.

7 The Hôpital des Quinze-Vingts, founded in 1260 by Louis IX.

8 Antonius Diogenes, *The Incredible Wonders Beyond Thule*, in Photius, *Biblioteca*, codice 166.

9 Herodotus, *Histories*, book 3, paragraph 116.

10 Virgil, *Æneid*, book 4, lines 165–6.

11 José de Acosta, *Historia natural y moral de las Indias* [Natural and Moral History of the Indies] (1590), book 7, chapter 22.

12 Virgil, *Eclogues*, book 8, line 41.

13 Ecclesiasticus (also known as the Book of Sirach), chapter 31, line 13.

14 Livy, *History of Rome*, book 26, chapter 22, lines 4–7.

15 Aristotle, *History of Animals*, book 6, chapter 18, lines 573b15–16.

www.ingramcontent.com/pod-product-compliance
Ingram Content Group UK Ltd.
Pitfield, Milton Keynes, MK11 3LW, UK
UKHW021033150926
475561UK00003B/86

9 781441 119322